I0100230

Ultimate Happiness

India Happiness Index is 140/156 as per UNO survey 2
Health is wealth. But wealth can't buy health and happ
Good health can lead to physical happiness. Wealth is ess
for life to run and happiness in life is dependent on
marriage, happy family and good social status. First we i
and spoil our health while earning wealth. Then we spe
wealth in regaining health. India is fast becoming capita
style diseases. Unhealthy person can't be happy. Spiritua
achieve happiness. We have to learn to be happy.

Ultimate Happiness

INDIA

Kartar S Birar

ZORBA BOOKS

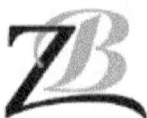

ZORBA BOOKS

Publishing Services by Zorba Books, 2019
Website: www.zorbabooks.com
Email: info@zorbabooks.com

Zorba Books Pvt. Ltd.(opc)
Gurgaon, INDIA

I dedicate this book to my dear and respected mother Shrimati Rama Devi who left for her heavenly abode at the age of eighty nine. She left us without any major sufferings and while living with us. She gave me my sense of humour.

Author

Acknowledgement

I would like to acknowledge and thank a very dear friend Colonel Achal Sridharan, who after premature retirement has established a brand 'Covai-Care', a new concept in Senior Living and Senior Care. I thought of senior citizen happiness after visiting his Coimbatore project and was inspired to write the book on Health, Wealth and Happiness.

I also thank my PA Mr. Naveen Kumar for type writing my hand written draft of this book for me to complete the book.

Author

Contents

Preface

Today India, as sixth largest economy in the world, fastest growing economy in the world, second most populous country and known as Land of spirituality, Nirwana, Moksha and Mukti but stands at serial 140 in happiness index among 156 countries surveyed by UNO. What are basics or fundamentals of happiness? These have been health, wealth, family life, social status and more than anything else the very sense of being happy and satisfied. Some call it sense of humour and satisfaction (santosham). What is most surprising in the happiness index is that we are behind China, Pakistan, Sri Lanka and USA. This position in the happiness index is going down every year in spite of our country growing economically upward. How can a country which is now becoming a capital of life style diseases like diabetes, cardio-vascular diseases and cancer, be happy? India has in last two decades, become a country where the overcrowding is found in number of big hospitals rather than in Gurudwaras, temples, mosques and Churches. Traditionally, Indians have been found in large crowds around religious cities/places. Our ancestors have been saying that basics of happiness or satisfaction state in a person's life are:-

- Health
- Wealth
- Family Life
- Social status/support
- State of Mind/Psychological Reasons

Our traditional couplet on happiness is as under:-

Pleasures of Life

First pleasure is good health,

Second pleasure is fair wealth.

Third pleasure spouse be loyal,

Fourth pleasure children are royal.

Fifth pleasure societal say,

Sixth pleasure peaceful home to stay.

Seventh pleasure at Guru's feet,

Eight pleasure God you meet.

जीवन के सुख

पहला सुख निरोगी काया

दूजा सुख घर में हो माया

तीजा सुख सतवंती नारी

चौथा सुख संतान आज्ञाकारी

पंचम सुख पंचों में पासा

षष्टम सुख शान्ति का बासा

सप्तम सुख सतगुरु के शरणम्

अष्टम सुख प्रभु के चरणम

अंतिम सुख धरती पर स्वर्ग

Some people think that one of the primary sources of happiness is money. But money cannot buy health and happiness. Some think retired life is full of problems and unhappiness. One of the greatest regrets of dying people is, "I wish I could have lived a little happier than what I have lived." As far as state of mind is concerned we are unhappy with life due to following reasons:-

- Unhappiness due to neighbours happiness.
- Negativity in perceptions like mother-in-Law and Daughter-in –Law relationship. If a daughter-in-law just thinks that her mother-in-law is mother of her husband for whom she has left her mother then there will be no unhappiness in their relationship.
- Grced, need and speed (Everything must get today)

I have completed seventy years and also completed fifteen years of retired life serving with three universities. I have tried to sum up my experiences with happiness in this book for my fellow citizens.

Author

Chapter – 1

Health is the Greatest Happiness

(Health is wealth)

A proverb.

Life Expectancy

The Bible says that your allotted years are three score and ten. The Vedas say that may you live for a century (Jeevan Shardhay Satam). Life expectancy in India has come a long way since forties. At the time of independence the average life expectancy was 32 years and today after 70 years or so it has reached 68 years. Of course, this cannot be taken as standard yard stick for planning your retired life. Approx 80% retired people in India live up to 75 years and remaining 20% live short and beyond this span. We, therefore, will accept 80 years to be the average life span and plan out our retired period accordingly. It is also pertinent that life expectancy in general, in India, may go higher in another decade or so.

Normal retirement age in govt jobs in our country spans from 56 to 60 years and in civil it spreads from 55 to 70 years. It will, therefore, be correct, if we presume that on an average residual life of 20 to 25 years after retirement need to be planned out. I have accepted this bracket of 20 to 25 years for the purpose of planning various activities before and after retirement. If you are lucky, you may even live up to one hundred years but if you are luckier then you may die at 75 or 80 years without any major illness or sufferings.

Health

Physical and mental health, after retirement, is by and large, important factors for any one and rest everything comes after health. If you have kept good or normal health so far then you may be lucky to maintain it. Generally, health deteriorates after sixty years and especially after the retirement. It is, therefore, very important to keep your body and mind busy and occupied as well, even after retirement.

As regards physical health, I would like to emphasise the importance of not gaining weight, after forty years or so majority of us gain weight due to lack of diet control and physical exercise. Fat or baby fat may be fabulous up to 16 years or so but after that it is a curse and also the cause of many serious and deadly diseases like hypertension, diabetes, coronary heart disease and the like. The ideal weight for a retired person (above 50 years) should be as given below:

Man		Woman	
Height (cms)	Weight (kgs)	Height (cms)	Weight (kgs)
156	55	150	43
158	56	152	44
160	57	154	44.5
162	58-59	156	45
164	60-61	158	46

Man		Woman	
Height (cms)	Weight (kgs)	Height (cms)	Weight (kgs)
166	62	160	47
168	64	162	49
170	65/66	164	51
172	67	166	52
174	68	168	54
176	70/71	170	56
178	72/73		
180	73/74		
182	75		
184	76		
186	78		
188	80		

Remember: Excess weight or obesity is number one enemy of health.

What is important to remember is that looking 'Mota Taza' is a mother's way of looking at health when you are school going kid? After that it is lean and famished look which is considered acceptable and in some other ways 'slim and trim' is also considered more sexy or smart as compared to fat and flabby looks. Two important factors which have a direct bearing on your weight are diet and physical exercise.

Calorie Count or Diet Control

The basic concept of diet intake should change after 35 years of age. You can afford to have good or rich food only if you have the will and capacity to digest it, otherwise it will add to your girth, belly or thighs. The basic philosophy of diet should be:-

- Eat to live and not live to eat.
- "Jaisa khaye ann whaisa ho tann aur mann."
  (Your body becomes what you eat)
- Every calorie must be counted.
- What is tasty for your tongue may not be good for your stomach and health.
- Eat three fourth or your hunger.
- Eat your meals as medicine otherwise you will eat medicine like your meals. Simply meaning quantity, quality and regularity for meals.

If you are a vegetarian then it's an added advantage. Otherwise you should become a vegetarian. In the West and US more and more people are turning towards vegetarianism. It may be pertinent to mention that eighty percent of non vegetarian items like meat, chicken, fowl and fish sold in the Indian markets are not even inspected by any one for any major disease. Would you, therefore, like to eat that stuff?

What to Eat

By the time you reach the stage of retirement you would have developed and patronized your tastes and menu. Some of us become very finical about our food and the way it should be prepared and served. I would suggest that we should bring in simplicity in our food habits and eat normal diet to say "Dal, Sabzi and Roti/Bhat". Fruits should be added and, if possible, one complete meal should be based on sprouts, salad and fruits. This could, ideally, be the breakfast. Lunch should be the main meal consisting of cereals, vegetables, curd and salad. Dinner should generally be light with soup, boiled vegetables and a little (150 ml) milk. In fact the good old saying of organizing your three meals should be:-

- Eat breakfast like a king.
- Eat lunch like a prince.
- And eat dinner like a pauper.

Should Avoid

- Three Ss i.e.; Sweets (sugar) Salt and Saturated fats.
- Heavy non vegetarian meals.
- Fried foods and fried snacks.
- Excessive alcoholic drinks and aerated drinks.
- Four Cs- Cakes, Candy, Cola and Chips.
- (These are generally known as junk food.)

Should Include

- Fibrous food and vegetables.
- Four Cs – Carrot, Cabbage, Cucumber and Capsicum. Incidentally these Cs take care of the Big 'C' i.e; (Cholesterol)
- Curd and cottage cheese in moderate quantities.
- Fruits, specially seasonal and citrus fruits.
- Nimboo paani should become your drink for the day and night.

Calorie Count

It will be very difficult to quantify the food intake as it would depend upon body weight, age and stomach size (hunger) developed over the last fifty-sixty years or so. It is, therefore, recommended that you should generally eat three fourth of your appetite. Whatever fruits or salads which cannot be chewed due to poor dental health or old age should be grated and consumed. In order to give a fair idea on calories, appetite and stomach size, it can be stated that a person of 55-60 years of age requires approx 2000 to 2500 calories depending upon the body weight and age. As you grow beyond sixty then approx 50 calories intake be reduced every two years.

A suggested daily menu for a person of 70 Kgs of weight and 60 years of age with normal health is as given below:-

Breakfast

- Unfried sprouts – one cup.
- Fruit (one banana or mango or apple or two oranges)
- Curd - one cup or 150ml of milk.

OR

- One roti of maize or bason with one glass of lassi (Buttermilk) or one cup of curd.
- Fruit as above.
- Black tea with fresh lemon.

OR

- Two Idlis.
- Cup of curd.

- Fruit as above.
- Black tea with fresh lemon.

OR

- Omelet without yellow one egg.
- Two toasts of whole wheat.
- One cup of milk with 20 gms of corn flakes.
- Black tea with fresh lemon.

Lunch

- Rotis made out of 100 gms of Atta or 50 gms plain cooked rice.
- Dal one cup.
- Vegetables (150 gms)
- Curd one cup/Lassi 150 gms. } Prepared in minimum Refined oil.
- Salad (100 gms).

Dinner/Supper

- Vegetable or Dal soup – 100 cc
- Boiled vegetable 200 gms.
- Chapatti/toasts one/two.
- Milk 100 cc (without fat i.e, skimmed)

In order to keep a count of your calories and substitute for high calorie items, which will be handy in calculating your intake, is given below:-

Vegetables and Fruits

For this	Calories	Substitute this	Calories	Calories Saved
VEGETABLES				
Potato (Fried), 1 Cup	450	Potato (Baked), 1 Cup	100	350
Potato (Mashed), 1 Cup	245	Potato (Boiled), 1 Cup	83	162
Peas, (Fresh), 100 gms	109	French beans, 100 gms	30	79
Brinjal (Cooked), 100 gms	69	Pumpkin (Cooked), ½ Cup	33	36
Onion (fresh), 1	45	Tomato (fresh), 1	20	25
Tomatoes (Stuffed & baked)	58	Tomato Slices (baked), 4	39	19
Corn (Baked), 1	64	Cabbage (Shredded)	12	52
Carrot (Fresh), 1	45	Cucumber (Fresh)	12	33
FRUITS				
Banana, 1	132	Apple, 1	56	76
Mango, 1	122	Melon, ½	37	85
Grapes, 22-24	70	Plum, 1	30	40
Pomegranate 100 gms	90	Papaya, 1/3	32	58
Pear, 1	64	Pineapple, 1 slice	44	40

For this	Calories	Substitute this	Calories	Calories Saved
Grape fruit, ½ medium	72	Peach, 1	50	22
Dates, 100 gms	283	Orange, 1	68	215

Sweet and Desserts

For this	Calories	Substitute this	Calories	Calories Saved
SWEETS & DESSERTS				
Jalebi, 100 gms	494	Gulab Jamun, 2	387	107
Rice Carrot Kheer, 100 gms	226	Rice Kheer, 100 gms	141	85
Sohan Halwa, 100 gms	399	Atta Halwa, 100 gms	263	136
Gujia, 100 gms	501	Maalpuwa, 100 gms	325	176
Cake (with icing), 1 piece	302	Cake (without icing), 1 piece	218	83
Pie (Fruit), 1(10 gms)	377	Baked Apple, 1	80	297
Butter Cookies, 100 gms	482	Mile Biscuits,100 gms	399	83
Boondi laddu, 1	150	Sandesh, 1	57	93
Custard (baked), 1 serving	250	Jelly, 1 serving	65	140

For this	Calories	Substitute this	Calories	Calories Saved
Pudding, 1 serving	50	Fruit salad 100 gms	80	105
Honey, 1 tsp	421	Sugar (Granular)	20	44
Jaggery, 1 tsp	348	Sugar (cube), 1tsp	24	32
FRUITS & OILS				
Groundnut oil, 1 tsp	126	Ghee, 1 tsp	45	81
Cream, 1 tsp	50	Butter, 1 tsp	36	14
Khoya, 100 gms	421	Khoya (butter separated) 100 gms	206	215
Paneer, 100 gms	348	Cheese (cottage), 1 tsp	27	321
		Cheese (chadder), 1 tsp	111	237

Beverages and Snacks

For this	Calories	Substitute this	Calories	Calories Saved
BEVERAGES				
Tea (2 tsp cream & 2 tsp sugar)	100	Tea 1 vup (2 tsp mild 2 tsp sugar)	60	50

For this	Calories	Substitute this	Calories	Calories Saved
Coffee 1 cup (2 tsp cream & 2 tsp sugar) milk	110	Coffee 1 cup (2 tsp milk & 2 tsp sugar)	60	50
Buffalo, 1 cup	206	Milk cow (skimmed)/ Butter milk 1 cup	78/62	128/144
Milk cow, 1 cup	160	Milk Buffalo (skimmed) / Butter milk 1 cup	70/62	90/98
Alcohol, (Rum/ Whisky) 43 ml	105	Brandy (30 ml)/Beer (1 glass)	73/100	32/5
Soft drink, 1 bottle	85	Squash, 1 glass	69	16
SNACKS				
Kachori, 1	190	Samosa, 1	103	87
Patti, 1	201	Cutlet, 1	126	75
Potato Vada, 1	118	Dahivada, 1	83	35
Chatt, 100 gms	474	Bhelpuri, 100 gms	182	292
Potato chips 20 gms	108	Peanuts (roasted), 1tbs	86	22

Pulses and Cereals

For this	Calories	Substitute this	Calories	Calories Saved
PULSES				
Bengal gram (roast) 100 gms	369	Bengal gram (cooked) 100 gms	105	264
		Black gram (cooked) 100 gms	105	264
		Green gram (cooked) 100 gms	105	264
		Lentil gram (cooked) 100 gms	105	264
		Red gram (cooked) 100 gms	105	264
Masoor dal with Rice, 100 gms	188	Mixed pulses with 100 gms vegetables	88	100
CEREALS				
Wheat Paratha, 1	304	Wheat Poori, 1		
Bajra, Jowar chapatti, 1	108–106	Wheat chapatti, 1		
Rice (Boiled), 140 gms	238	Idli (Rice) 2 pieces		

For this	Calories	Substitute this	Calories	Calories Saved
Idli (Rice), 2 Pieces	130	Idli (Suji) 2 pieces		
Upama, 1 Plate (260 gms)	397	Sada Dosa, 1 (100 gms)		

Physical Activity

In order to keep your muscles toned, burn calories which you have consumed and maintain your cardio-vascular system in good state, it is important that you maintain a fair amount of regular physical activity. Five golden rules in this sphere are:-

- Health is wealth.
- Healthy body – sound mind.
- Rest more than eight hours is the surest formula for rusting.
- Use it lose it.
- Keep sitting on a chair and table, you tend to become a vegetable.

It is, therefore, very important to have some regular physical activity in the form of brisk walking, jogging, cycling, swimming and some simple aerobics to maintain good health. It is commonly believed that as you become a senior citizen you tend to lose interest in sex. Some even go further and recommend that you should practice celibacy after retirement. Doctors and sexologists opine that healthy sexual activity is an excellent form of aerobic exercise. Approximately 120-150 calories are burnt and in this aspect "Bhoga is superior to Yoga". I am not, by any chances decrying the established science of Yoga. 'Yoga Abhayas requires guidance, and supervision from a trained teacher and far greater time and dedication. If you have developed a hobby like golf or gardening then this will definitely prove useful during this phase of life. Ideal physical exercise for a retired person is long (5-6 km) morning walk followed up by mild and simple aerobic exercises like side jump, bending and stretching for 15-20 minutes. A lot will, of course, depend upon the place of residence and facilities available there in.

Calories Burnt

A man of 175 cms height and weighing 70 kgs is likely to burn calories during physical activity as under:-

- Walking at 4 kmph – 6 calories per minute.
- Jogging at 12 kmph – 20 calories per minute.
- Cycling at 10 kmph – 10 calories per minute.
- Swimming continuously – 12 calories per minute.
- Reclining – 1.5 calories per minute.

After these exercises for one hour or so, you should take aerobics followed by long breaths for about 15–20 minutes, standing with legs one meter apart or laying down on your back. A simple calorie count formula is to burn calories equal to calories consumed. This will facilitate maintaining well toned muscles and body weight. If your intake of calories is more than what you can burn, you will gain weight and vice versa.

Therefore, remember "calories intake should be equal to or less than calories burnt".

Calories intake < Calories burnt

A suggested daily routine with time chart has been included in a chapter later, on hobby and pastime.

Conclusion

There is a famous saying on health

- If wealth is lost then nothing is lost.
- If health is lost then something is lost.
- If reputation/Character is lost then everything is lost.

Chapter – 2

Preventive Health

(Prevention is better than cure)

Yoga as Best Preventive Medicine

Yoga and Ayurved are our greatest medical and health treasure from time immemorial. Swami Ramdev Ji has marketed this to millions of house hold as practicing ambassador in 21st century. If he had not done this then things by now would have been different. May be a blonde from USA would have been teaching Yoga in Indian Yogashrams.

Swami Ramdev Ji says "Karo Yog, Raho Nirog". He has, in the last 20 years of his effort to take the yoga to lakhs of households in our country, demonstrated and proved that 'Yoga including Pranayams' are the best preventive and social medicine in the field of preventive, pro-motive and social medicine. He has personally conducted more than three thousand camps of seven days and short camps (3–4days). He has travelled 11 lakhs Km, trained more the ten lakh people and helped in improving health of more than ten lakh people with Yoga and Pranayam. All these records are maintained in Patanjali Yogpeeth.

This chapter briefly describes the daily yoga regime specially designed for senior citizen. The chapter also contains a brief on yoga as philosophy of life and how it can bring efficiency and full coordination of Body-Mind-Soul combination.

Scientific Package of 12 Asanas and 8 Pranayams (One hour 15 Mins) Sequence

1. Warming up- 5 mins
2. Asanas (12), 25 mins → Mandook Asans
3. Sitting Position Asan → Shashak Asans
   Cow Mouth Vakrasan

4. Lying on Stomach Position → Makrasan Shalabh asan
   Bhujang asan
   Dhanur asan

5. Lying on Back Position → Markat asan- 4 elements
   Pawan Mukatasan-I & II
   Ardh Hal Asan
   Div Chakra Asan

6. Shav Asan 2–3 mins = 33 mins
7. Pranayam
   - (i) Bhastrika : 5 mins
   - (ii) Kapal Bhati : 15 mins
   - (iii) Bahya : 3 mins
   - (iv) Ujjayi : 2 mins
   - (v) Anulom Vilom : 5 mins
   - (vi) Bhrameri : 5 mins

(vii)	Chanting of Om	:	1 mins
(viii)	Pranav	:	1 mins
	Total		**= 45 mins**

Grand Total = 45 + 33 = 78 mins. The detailed description of these is given at the end of this book with photographs.

What is Yoga?

'Yoga' is a Sanskrit word meaning 'to add' or addition. One may ask 'to add' what and with whom? The answer is very simple, to add 'Atman 'to 'Parmatman'. With the regime of yoga practice it is aimed to connect your body to good health and your Atma to Parmatma.

'Yoga' is also an acronym for '**Your Own Godly Awareness**'. If a person follows the principles of yoga sincerely and completely then the regime of 'Yoga and Pranayama' can take him to a stage of self awareness or realization. Though the acronym is in English language but it is true in Hindi meaning also.

'Yoga' is also described as regime of efficiency, efficacy and entirety. In our Holy Geeta, Lord Krishna has called Yoga as "**Yoga Karmeshu Kauhalam**" meaning yoga as harbinger of efficiency in all actions of human being.

Maharishi Patanjali has written in his Yoga Sutra, "**Yog Chittvarti Nirodhah**". Yoga causes stability of mind and removes all vices from the psyche of a person.

There are thousands of Granthas, Sutras, Sanhitas and Shashtra where a lot has been written about yoga by different

Rishis, Munis and Yoga Acharyas. Yoga is a real hidden treasure of our ancient culture and civilization. Lord Shiva is considered to be first Guru of "Yoga" and his disciples (Shisyas) are supposed to be Mata Parvati, Rishi Machhander and Gorakhnath. The original and authenticated yoga texts are found in the following sources:-

- Bhagvad Geeta.
- Shiv Sanhita.
- Patanjali Yoga Sutra.
- Gherand Sanhita.
- Hath Yoga Pradeepika.
- Vedas, Upnishads and Purans.

Types of Yoga

Yogas are performed in many ways. Some of these important and prevalent ones are:-

Karam Yoga	**Dhayan Yoga**	**Laya Yoga**
Shankhay Yoga	**Gyan Yoga**	**Hath Yoga**
Sanyas Yoga	**Raj Yoga**	**Tarang Yoga**
Bhakti Yoga	**Mantra Yoga**	**Swar Yoga**
Astang Yoga	**Tantar Yoga**	**Sahaj Yoga**

It may be relevant to give a short explanation of each or them to understand simple meaning of these forms of yoga. Yoga Philosophy (Yog Darshan) is one of the six important philosophies of life in India.

Karam and Sankhya Yoga:- Theses two types of yoga have been described in detailed in chapter 2 and 3 of Bhagvad Geeta. This simply means getting addicted to your "duty and knowledge of self". You do your duty and know yourself like a yogi performing his yoga. The sincerity and knowledge of performing the duty without waiting for the fruits or results is the ultimate purpose of Karama and Sankhya yoga.

Sanyas yoga & Moksha Sanyas Yoga:- The ultimate purpose of the yoga is to attain Moksha or Nirvana while performing yoga as Sanyas or in Sanyas Asharam.

Gyan & Dhayan Yog:- The aim of this yoga is to practice meditation and attain self knowledge and knowledge of Parmatma.

Raj Yoga:- The aim is to perform your duty as dharma while enjoying all gift of God.

Bhakti Yoga:- The aim is to perform Bhakti (Japp, Tapp, Recitation and meditation) and attain Moksha.

Many other types of yoga are:-

- Sangeet Yoga-Music Yoga.
- Sahaj Yoga-Simply meditating.
- Lahar Yoga-Wave therapy or yoga.
- Mantra Yoga-A regime of Mantras.
- Tantra Yoga-A regime of Tantrik Mantras.
- Swar Yoga-meaning Swar (recitation) yoga.

Hath Yoga:- A form of Astang yoga with concentration on awakening of Kundalini shakti.

Astang Yoga:- Astang yoga is a regime of yoga which has eight parts (astang). These eight parts have a special sequence and each part has its own subparts. These eight parts are:-

- Yama (Self control, in behavior with others)
- Niyam (Self control and social norms)
- Asana (A regime and sequence of body postures which are totally scientific)
- Pranayam (A regime and sequence of breathing exercises based on scientific approach)
- Pratyahar (Detachment from worldly vices, pleasure and Maya)
- Dharna (withdrawing all senses into self and bringing stability and concentration.)
- Dhayan (Meditation and self realization)
- Samadhi (Connecting Atman (Soul) to Paramtma (God) or Realisation of self and God.

Astang yoga is the most practiced most prevalent, most adopted and most scientific for body, mind and soul. How each of these parts control different parts of human being is shown by a diagram below:-

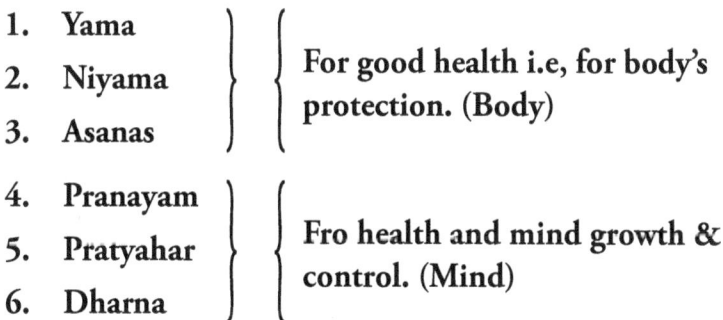

1. **Yama**
2. **Niyama** } { **For good health i.e, for body's protection. (Body)**
3. **Asanas**

4. **Pranayam**
5. **Pratyahar** } { **Fro health and mind growth & control. (Mind)**
6. **Dharna**

7. **Dhayan**
8. **Samadhi** } { **For body-mind control and spiritual growth. (Soul)**

This sequence of Astang Yoga and regular practice makes a person:-

- Physically fit.
- Mentally alert.
- Emotionally balanced.
- Socially adept and accepted.
- Rationally positive.
- Spiritually elevated.
- Detached from all vices.
- Self analytic.
- Self aware.
- Self realized leading to God realization.

A brief description of eight parts of Astang Yoga is given below.

1. Yama:- Comprises of five sub elements, these are, 1. Non-violence, 2. Truth, 3. Non stealing, 4. Celibacy and 5. Non hoarding. While ser 1 to 3 and ser 5 are well understood, ser 4 i.e. celibacy for a married man may cause little confusion. It means controlled derives, relationship and sex only with complete consent. It may be difficult to lay down any frequency but should suffice to say that excess of everything including sex is bad. Infact the real word for a married person is continence rather than complete celibacy.

2. Niyama:- This also comprises of five elements. These are- 1. Cleanliness, 2. Satisfaction, 3. Penance, 4. Self Study, 5. Surrender to the God. The simplest explanations of these Niyama are:

- Cleanliness is next to Godliness.
- Satisfaction brings happiness (Ananda)
- Penance brings Moksha.
- Self –Study brings (Gyana)
- Surrender to God causes ultimate love and union with God.

3. Asanas:- It's a regime of body postures with proper sequence, frequency and duration for each asana. The details about these are given at the end of this book.

4. Pranayam:- It simply means a set of breathing exercises with proper duration, sequence and frequency. This will also be explained in a subsequent chapter. Basically it comprises three events i.e. breathing in i.e. inhalation, holding of breath and breathing out i.e. exhaling.

5. Pratyahar:- This is the last external sequence for body and brain. This amounts to drawing all your five senses inward and detaching them from external environment for further progress towards Dharna.

6. Dharna (Concentration):- The process of drawing yourself inward and concentrating toward inner mind so that you can further meditate towards inner journey.

7. Dhayan (Meditation):- The process of attaching yourself with inward journey is called Dhayan or meditation.

8. Samadhi (Union):- The ultimate goal of yoga is to unite Atma (Soul) with Parmatma (God) and this union is called Samadhi. When a person does everything for and sake of God then it is called perfect union. It is also meant that when a person reaches the stage of Egolessness then Samadhi is achieved. It is the ultimate goal of life and with Samadhi you achieve 'Moksha' or 'Nirvana' or libration or Jannat. Swami Satyanada Sarswati has written in his book 'Meditation from Tantras:- "All forms of yoga aim at bringing about the state of meditation. One type of yoga should not be practiced to the exclusion of all others. Though they are usually regarded as the different paths of yoga, a more realistic description would be to call yoga the path, and its different forms the different lanes of that path. This can be compared to a piece of rope composed of various smaller strands. The different strands have separate identities, yet together they form the rope. In the same way be different strands of each type of yoga, when performed in conjunction with each other, form the composite whole which takes one to meditation."

Yog literally means to add or to connect. In this way we can say that yog connects:-

Body	$\longrightarrow$	Good health and karma
Mind	$\longrightarrow$	Gyan/Knowledge
Mann	$\longrightarrow$	Karma/Purushartha
Chitt	$\longrightarrow$	Guru
Atman	$\longrightarrow$	Paramatman

Normal Problems of Senior Citizens

As the age advances and the bones & muscles in the body begin to degenerate and some of the normal problems occur generally after 50 years of age. There are:-

- Low back ache (LBA) or back pain.
- Joint pain in the entire body.
- Shoulder freezing.
- Sciatica Nerve pain.
- Cervical Spondylitis.

In addition to these bones and muscular problems some nervous/psychiatric i.e. brain related problems also regularly adopted as normal way of life and a correct diet and drink regime is adopted, then these problems can be mostly avoided. In order to clearly diagnose and come to real problems annual/six monthly medical checkup is recommended. A visit to medical specialist, orthopaedician and psychiatrist is recommended in case the problems continue to persist.

The aim here is to give you a specific preventive and promotive Yog regime which can prevent and control these ailments. Any joint in the body is made of bones, cartelizes, ligaments joint fluids and muscles. It would be our aim to recommend such Asanas and Pranayams to prevent these ailments and help a person to handle these ailments in addition to preventive measures.

Low back Ache (LBA):-

Spine is like the central pillar of the body and it holds the body weight and also holds it erect. In addition to inter vestibular joints the dorsal muscles weakening could be a cause of LBA. There could be many more causes of back ache (LBA) and these are:-

- Fair wear and tear of body, muscles and bones.
- Slip disc or IVDP (Inter Vestibular Disc Prolapse).
- Improper method of sitting, standing, walking or lifting of weight etc.
- Any jerk shock or trauma causing muscular spasm.
- Osteophytes.
- Osteoporosis.
- Normal Arthritis.
- Irregular life routine.
- Improper sleeping habits.
- Poor life style with poor diet.
- Lack of exercise, yog or any other work out.
- Ladies can experience LBA, due to periodic cycle or excessive bleeding.
- Many other causes which must be diagnosed if the problem persists.

Preventive Measures:

- Always stand erect on both legs.
- Do regular 5 km walk.
- Sit with spine erect.
- Be careful while bending and lifting.
- Sleep on a hard bed.
- Breathe normally through your nostrils.

- Do not allow weight increase.
- Do not ignore any indication of LBA and do not allow it to increase.
- Do not overstretch and exert.
- Do not cause any jerk/pull.
- Do not force any movement beyond you can comfortably do.
- Do not perform yogas if you are suffering from any other medical problems.

Yoga Asan Recommended:

- Warming up exercise like bending sideways, for ward & rear.
- Surya Namaskar at normal pace(two cycles per minutes)
- Maker Asan.
- Bhujang Asan.
- Markat Asan.
- Gau Mukh Asan. (Cow Mouth)
- Dhanur Asan.
- Butter Fly Asan.

Joint Pain:

Causes could be on the same lines as also how back ache. However, in most cases joint pain occurs due to old age and arthritis. A regular life style and routine can cause delay in setting of joint pain. Basically all the joints of the body must be exercised in the direction they are supposed to function. Right from hand fingers, wrist joint, elbow joint shoulder joint, vestibular exercises and lower limbs including ankle and toes should be exercised daily in a proper sequence i.e. from top to bottom or bottom to top. In addition the daily package of 12 Asanas and Pranayams should be practiced daily.

Shoulder Freezing:

Shoulder joint like any other joint of the body should also be exercised daily. As the age grows the use of shoulder joint for lifting or any other work reduces tremendously. Most shoulder freezing takes place due to non use of the joint and other reasons as in case of arthritis. Shoulder joint should be exercised by rotating, lifting and strengthening exercise daily. Along with this Gaumukh Asan should be practiced daily, at least twice a day, for 2–3 minutes.

Sciatica Pain:

Sciatic Nerve is thickest and longest nerve in the human body. It originates from brain and ends at the heels and divides into two at the lumber region. Any pressure on this nerve, any pull or jerk or any stretch while lifting or any accidental shock can cause Sciatica nerve pain. One of the best methods to take care is to relax and do soft messages and movements. Pain killer tablets should be avoided, however, application of gels and pain relieving oils are recommended.

Asans Recommended

- Makar Asan.
- Vakra Asan.
- Butter Fly Asan.
- Baby swing with folded leg.

Sciatica pain normally subsides after a week or so. Rest, soft movements, slow and steady Asans will provide good enough relief. Soft messages and pain relieving gels should be used.

Cervical Spondylitis:

Neck muscles are special type of muscles and if these are not exercised well or abused i.e. improperly used then this problem can occur. The weight of the head is supported by seven cervical vertebras. If neck muscles are week then pressure is caused on the nerves which cause very severe pain. It is possible to prevent this problem by:-

- Regular neck exercises.
- Proper sleeping habits.
- Use of normal i.e. 4 to 5 inches pillow.
- Proper sitting, standing and walking maintaining neck posture.
- Avoiding long office hours and use of low table or bending of neck very low.

In case of this problem occurs and persists then cervical collar after advice form a surgeon is the answer.

100 Benefits of Meditation

Meditation should be practiced at least twice a day. Once in the morning with the Yog Regime and once in the evening. Evening Meditation with Guru Mantra or Om Chanting can be done before going to bed. It helps in giving good sleep.

I. Physiological benefits

1. It lowers oxygen consumption.
2. Decreases respiratory rate.
3. Increases blood flow and slow the heart rate.
4. Increases exercise tolerance.
5. Leads to a deeper level of physical relaxation.
6. Good for people with high blood pressure.
7. Reduces anxiety attacks by lowering the levels of blood lactate.
8. Decreases muscle tension.
9. Helps in chronic diseases like allergies, arthritis etc.
10. Reduce pre-menstrual symptoms.
11. Helps in post-operative healing.
12. Enhances the immune system.
13. Reduces activity of viruses and emotional distress.
14. Enhances energy, strength and vigour.
15. Helps with weight loss.
16. Reduction of free radicals, less tissue damage.
17. Higher skin resistance.
18. Drop in cholesterol levels, lower risk of cardiovascular diseases.
19. Improved flow or air to the lungs resulting in easier breathing.
20. Decreases the ageing process.
21. Higher level of (Dehydroepiandrosterone).
22. Prevents, slows or controls pain of chronic diseases.

23. Makes you sweat less

24. May help in curing headaches & migraines

25. Greater orderliness or brain functioning

26. Reduced need for medical care

27. Less energy wasted

28. More inclined to sports, activities

29. Significant relief from asthma

30. Improved performance in athletic events

31. Normalizes to your ideal weight

32. Harmonizes our endocrine system

33. Relaxes our nervous system

34. Produces lasting beneficial changes in brain electrical activity

35. May help in curing infertility (the stresses of infertility can interfere with the release of hormones that regulate ovulation)

II. Psychological Benefits

36. Builds self-confidence

37. Increase serotonin level, influences mood and behavior

38. Resolves phobias and fears

39. Helps control own thoughts

40. Helps with focus and concentration

41. Increases creativity

42. Increases brain wave coherence

43. Improved learning ability and memory

44. Increased feeling of vitality and rejuvenation

45. Increased emotional stability

46. Improved relationships

47. Mind ages at slower rate

48. Easier to remove bad habits

49. Develops intuition

50. Increased Productivity

51. Improved relations at home and work

52. Ability to see the larger picture in a given situation

53. Helps ignore petty issues

54. Increased ability to solve complex problems

55. Purifies your character

56. Develops will power

57. Greater communication between the two brain hemisphere

58. React more quickly and more effectively to a stressful event.

59. Increases one's perceptual ability and motor performance

60. Higher intelligence growth rate

61. Increased job satisfaction

62. Increases the capacity for intimate contact with loved ones

63. Decreases the potential for mental illness

64. More sociable behavior

65. Less aggressiveness

66. Helps in smoking cessation and alcohol addiction

67. Reduces the need and dependency on drugs, pills and pharmaceuticals

68. Less need of sleep to recover from sleep deprivation
69. Requires less time to fall asleep, helps to cure insomnia.
70. Increases sense of responsibility
71. Reduces road rage
72. Decreased in restless thinking
73. Decreased tendency to worry
74. Increases listening skills and empathy
75. Helps to make more accurate judgments
76. Greater tolerance
77. Gives composure to act in considered and constructive ways
78. Grows a stable, more balanced personally
79. Develops emotional maturity

III. Spiritual Benefits

80. Helps to keep things in perspective
81. Provides peace of mind, happiness
82. Helps to discover your purpose
83. Increased self-actualization
84. Increased compassion
85. Spiritual growth
86. Deeper understanding of yourself and others
87. Brings body, mind, spirit in harmony
88. Deeper level of spiritual relaxation
89. Increased acceptance of oneself
90. Helps to learn forgiveness

91. Changes attitude toward life

92. Creates a deeper relationship with your higher power or deity

93. Attains enlightenment

94. Greater inner-directedness

95. Helps living in the present moment

96. Creates a widening, deepening capacity for love

97. Discovery of the power and consciousness beyond the ego.

98. Experience an inner sense of assurance

99. Experience a sense of oneness

100. Increases the synchronicity in one's life

Asna & Pranayamas for Daily Regime

Basic Golden Rules

Senior citizen must follow the three basic golden rules of Asanas and Pranayams:-

- NO Force. You must feel comfortable.
- No Speed. You must follow normal speed.
- No Jerks. You must not do any act with a Jerk.

With these golden rules, you may take more than one and half to two hours in the beginning. Once you get into the rut/routine then you will take 1hr 20 minutes to follow the regime. For details of this regime please see the Appendix to this book.

Prevention is Better than Cure

Can we prevent ageing? May be, we can delay it! It seems, if we can prevent or curb disease in old age, thus this period of life can be made more satisfying, happy and worth living.

This brings us to the question: what brings on ageing? Many theories have been propounded in this regard. I would, however, like to quote a relevant passage from **Charaka Samhita**, an ancient Ayurvedic text. It states:

All ills of the body arise..... In consumer of sour, salt, pungent and alkaline articles, dried vegetables, flesh.... Softened, heavy, stale foods, meals taken at irregular times or in irregular quantities or too frequently, i.e., over a stomach that has not yet recovered from the last meal, addicts in day sleeping, sex pleasures and wine bibbing, persons whose bodies have been strained by fault or inordinate indulgence in exercise; and victims of fear, anger, grief, infatuation overwork...

Therefore, having regard to such ills, one should give up the above-mentioned unwholesome diet and regimen.

Features of Ageing

As you grow older, changes take place in body. These are:-

- External changes like loss of hair, wrinkles on face and skin, fat accumulation and unsteady posture.
- Internal changes in the working of digestive system, liver, pancreas, cardio-vascular system, lungs, kidneys, Central Nervous System and reproductive system.
- Weakening of sensory facilities like vision, hearing, smell, taste etc.

Some people look younger than their age, and some older. Some people have a longer life-span and other die at a much younger age. What are the causes that influence and the length of the life? A lot of research has been done on this topic. Actually, if I can say, everyone wants to **look younger and live longer**.

Some of the factors which affect ageing are:-

- Heredity
- Environment
- Climate and altitude
- Diet
- Physical activity
- Psycho-social factors
- Stress
- Disease

System of Medicines

From time immemorial, man has aspired for a long life, youthful vigour and good health. Different means have been used to attain this goal, prayers, use of herbals and minerals, exercise, yoga, and proper diet.

Some success, in this direction has been achieved. The life span of man has increased and some of the diseases have been eliminated/ reduced, making human life healthier, more productive and more worth living.

Let us now see how the different systems of medicine prevalent in India, set out to achieve it and how much they have contributed to it. Some of the methods used have been described from the original texts.

Ayurveda. The Indian system of medicine, by its very name means the "science of long life". Its concept of good health covers physical, mental, moral and spiritual fitness. Ayurveda has always given fullest attention to prevention of diseases and attaining healthy long life.

Naturopathy. Naturopathy's way to long life is through cooperating with nature to do its normal function. The primary cause of all diseases, according to Naturopathy, is the conscious or unconscious violation of Nature's laws. This may be in thinking, breathing eating, drinking, dressing, working, resting as well as in moral, social and sexual conduct.

Diseases in reality are a self-purifying effort on the part of Nature. Lindlahr states: "Every acute disease is the result of the cleaning and healing effect of Nature. If you suppress the acute conditions by drugs or by any other means, you are simply laying the foundation for chronic diseases. All diseases from a simple cold to skin eruptions, diarrhea, fever, etc..., represent Nature's effort to remove from the system some of the method or toxic matter, some poison dangerous to health and life.

In India, our religious texts like the Vedas and Upanishads, and the secular ones like those of Ayurveda, lay the greatest stress on living with Nature and making use of natural stimuli for promotion of health, longevity and cure of diseases.

In the last century, Gandhiji was one of the greatest enthusiasts of nature cure methods or naturopathy.

Naturopathy procedures accomplish this aim by assisting Nature in removing from the body the accumulated toxins. They stimulate the organs of elimination to better functioning and thus restore the diseased and disordered organs their normal tone, blood supply, glandular activity, etc. They also intend to bring back to normal, the abnormal physical and mental habits of the patient so as to stop further harm to the body and to teach him to live with the Nature and not against it.

The procedure which naturopathy recommends to be used in maintaining and restoring health is daily cleanliness, physical exercise, relaxation and regulation of diet. They also include the use in different forms of water, earth, air and sunshine. Some people also include under it measures such as massages and pressure point.

Yoga.   Yoga is not a system of medicine, yet through it, one can attain long life and a "sound mind in a sound body". According to Patanjali, the author of Yoga-sutras, Yoga, consists of eight components, viz., yama, niyama asana, pranayama, pratyahara, dharana, dhayana and Samadhi. The first four components relate more to the body; they prepare the body for the next four components which relate more to the mind and soul.

Unani System.   Unani medicine is built upon, the ancient Greek medical concepts of Hippocrates and Galen as conceived and expanded by al-Raz and ibn-Sina and other Arabic and Persian physicians. It makes use of herbs, minerals and animal products to keep the body fit and to promote long life.

Homeopathy.   Homeopathy as such does not claim to prolong life span except through treatment of diseases and thereby restoring health. According to Hahnemann, the founder of the system, human body functions and is maintained by a vital force. This force is capable of adjusting the body and mind to the best advantage of the person when he is threatened by adverse influences. Diseases mean disorderly functioning of this vital force. In acute disease, this vital force though disordered to a great extent or even to the point of extinction, still retains an inherent capacity to set itself right with or without medicinal help. In chronic diseases, however, the vital force though altered in an insidious way gets so deranged that it seems to have lost that inherent capacity or self-adjustment.

When a patient responds to treatment, according to Homoeopathic concept, his complaints shift form one area of the body to another, usually from more vital organs to less vital organs, as if some inner healing force were directing their course. Head symptoms move down towards the trunk and gradually along the extremities to the hands and feet. Illness or vital organs such as the lungs and heart would shift into the throat or intestine may be ending as a discharge or as a skin eruption. Mental illnesses would move into the emotional and then into the physical sphere. In the case of a long standing disease under treatment, the most recent symptoms that the patient had will reappear for a brief period first, and the oldest symptoms, the last.

Under Homeopathy, the symptoms of illness are often not considered dangerous in themselves to be removed by any means, but instead they represent an attempt by the body to heal itself. Behind every symptom of a particular illness is the attempt of the body to restore balance.

Living with the nature, and using the minimum quantities of medicines, when needed, so as to reactivate the vital force of the body, brings about, according to Homoeopathy, good health, freedom from disease and consequently long life.

Modern Medicine. (Allopathy) Avoidance of ill-health, curing diseases and thus prolonging life, has been practiced through Western (now modern) medicine since the time of Hippocrates of Galen.

Animal experiments conducted so far indicate that all efficacious pharmacological therapies show their effects by a reduction of disease vulnerability and not by a decrease of ageing rate.

Making man immortal is against the law of nature. Good health and long-life are as much a gift of nature as they are the results or one's own efforts of a balanced life style, keeping in view the role of diet, physical exercise and a spirit of "live and let live".

Why Prevention?

Dr OP Jaggi in his book "Health Care for Plus Fifty" narrates details about ageing and prevention. He says "when an older person falls ill, there are some features which are more often met because of the age and not because of a particular disease. These have to be recognized and sorted out from the particular features of a disease, so as to manage the whole patient as best as possible".

Some of the reasons are:-

(a) **Multiple Pathology**. In old age, it is a rule rather than the exception for the patient to suffer from several diseases at a time. In an acute illness, it is usually clear which diseases are dominate, but some other ailments also must be taken into account.

A patient with a brain stroke, for example, may well be handicapped, also be cataract which limits his vision, heart disease which limits his capacity, a urinary infection which increases the risk of incontinence, and osteo-arthritis of this hips or knees which further limits his mobility. All these as well as the stroke, demand treatment and influence his rehabilitation.

(b) **Tendency of Confusion**. In case of an old man, the stability of the brain is precariously balanced, probably because of the loss of nerve cells which accompany ageing. The function of the brain is readily upset by and kind of bodily disturbance and a sudden onset of confusion is one of the commonest indications of physical illness in old age. In a patient without previous mental impairment, the onset of confusion suggests serious physical illness, but in those whose minds are already beginning to fail, confusion may be provoked by quite minor bodily disturbances. Such reactions are often short-lived and subside as soon as the physical disorder is corrected.

(c) **Lesser Sensibility to Pain.** An old man often has a diminished sense of pain. This makes life less uncomfortable for him, but it increases the risk that he may injure himself. For example, he may burn his shins by sitting too close to the fire. Hot water bottles are a special danger. Even serious injuries like fractures may not be obvious. An old person, who breaks the neck of his femur, may have only mild discomfort even though he cannot walk. In acute abdominal conditions such as acute appendicitis, there may be little pain or tenderness until the disease is far advanced and the patient is gravely ill.

(d) **Diminished Temperature Regulation.** The regulation of body temperature is less efficient in the older patient and fever is less obvious and less severe. Thus an illness which would provoke a sharp rise in temperature in a younger patient, may in the elderly cause only a small rise or none at all. If an old person seems unwell, there can be no reassurance in the fact that his temperature is normal. The pulse and respiration are often a better guide to his condition. The defective temperature regulation of the older patient is also seen in his reaction to cold when his body temperature falls far below normal in the condition known as hypothermia.

(e) **Reaction of Drugs.** An older patient is very sensitive to drugs and harmful side–effects are common. Drugs are more slowly metabolized in the liver and because of diminished renal function, take longer to excrete. Thus medicines should be given in smaller doses. For example, digoxin is effective in one-quarter of the dose used for younger people. The margin of error in prescribing between the dose which does well and the overdose which may harm must be understood. Moreover, one drug may react with another in unexpected ways and the multiple diseases often present, may mean that several drugs are needed. The precarious stability of the brain makes confusion a common side–effect of many drugs.

(f) **Fatigue.** Persistent or recurrent fatigue is a common symptom in older patients. It is to be expected in wasting illnesses generally, but it should also suggest a search for anemia of gradual onset. It is a prominent symptom in heart disease, in which it may be complained of as much as breathlessness. It accompanies congestive heart failure, and states of low blood pressure, but in particular, left ventricular failure and cases of coronary artery disease in which the heart is enlarged and close to failing.

(g) **Sleep Disturbance.** An older person's sleep is often interrupted by aches and pains of various kind, especially rheumatic pain, the distressing ischemic pain of peripheral vascular diseases affecting the feet and legs, leg cramps, and above all, by the need to urinate at night. The latter is not uncommon even in the absence of bladder or kidney diseases or diabetes. Most insomnia is a consequent of various discomforts. In the presence of anxiety, there is usually some difficulty in falling sleep at night; with depression, the tendency is for the patient to wake up early and to toss and turn in the bed. Both these disorders are common in elderly people.

(h) **Loss of Appetite.** If the illness is of a toxic or pyrexial nature, old patients lose their appetite completely and are content to exist for day or weeks on fluids only. Appetite is probably the last thing to recover too.

(i) **Breathlessness.** Breathlessness may be due to disorders of the lungs, heart, and blood and so on. An older patient may have periodic respiration wherein he stops breathing at all for some seconds, before resuming normal rhythm. This may appear very alarming to the attendants.

(j) **Vertigo.** A complaint of giddiness or dizziness is one the commonest symptoms among the elderly. These are subjective sensations that are always unpleasant and sometimes frightening. They indicate instability of posture, some immediate spatial disorientation, and in severe forms a sensation or rotation and extreme distress.

Some Additional Hazards

Young people get over their illness because of ample bodily reserves which helps them to fight them. Older people have fewer reserves and so run the risk of various complications of their illness that are not usually expected in younger individuals. Thus, a young person may be immobilized for long periods without coming to any harm, but an older person deteriorates fast in general mobility and capability, in vigour and even in spirit if he cannot move about. This happens more so in those who are already arthritic or have disorders of mobility.

Confinement to bed for older people is a harbinger of a bagful or problems. Those commonly seen are constipation, incontinence of urine and faces, pressure sores, contractures of the joints, bed sores and thrombo-embolism.

Preventive Health Care

Drug Administration

Ageing causes changes in the body with regard to drug absorption, distribution and action. It is important to understand this changed behavior of the body towards drugs so that a proper response is obtained, and side-effects eliminated or diminished.

Factors Influencing Drug Response

(a) **Absorption.** Following their absorption, all drugs pass in the abdominal circulation to the liver where some undergo substantial metabolism before entering the general circulation, a phenomenon known as the first-pass effect.

A reduction in liver metabolic activity is likely to be reflected in a reduced first-pass effect and increased systemic bioavailability following oral administration of the drug.

(b) **Distribution.** The age-related decline of serum albumin concentration produces significant increase in unbound plasma concentration of several drugs that are strongly bound to protein (e.g., salicylates, sulfadiazine and phenylbutazone). The adverse effect of corticosteroids occurs more frequently in patients with low serum albumin concentration.

(c) **Metabolism.** The enzyme system in the liver is the major site of drug metabolism. There is an overall tendency for the metabolic activity of the older individuals to be less efficient than in the youth.

(d) **Excretion.** For some drugs, e.g, antibiotics like streptomycin, and digoxin, the kidney is the major route of elimination. Changes in renal function associated with ageing have important implications for such drugs. The elderly are at risk of reduced clearance and resulting accumulation of the parent drug and the active metabolites.

(e) **Action Response.** Response of the body to drugs depends on their action on target tissues and organs. This ultimately reflects the ability of the free or unbound concentration or the drug to react with specific cell or its parts, and to initiate specific action. That action is modified by factors such as homeostatic control mechanisms, the influence of disease state and concurrent medications.

Is the Drug Really Needed?

With increasing number of older patients and with increasing diagnosis of common disorders such as hypertension and old age (maturity-onset) diabetes, it is critical that we optimize our therapeutic strategies. There is little doubt that elevated blood pressure and bold glucose levels contributes to morbidity and mortality in all age-groups. However, the evidence is far from clear that the normalization by drugs of either blood pressure or blood glucose in entirely asymptomatic patients, contributes to improved longevity, reduced morbidity or a more desirable quality of life in the older patient.

Surgery

Three types of situations arise in the elderly with regard to surgery.

First, where there is no choice and the surgery has to be done as an emergency, as example, in case of intestinal obstruction.

Second, where the operation has to be done, but it is not an emergency, as for example, prostate removal. Here there is time to plan an operation and if there are some risk factors in the patient, they can be corrected or improved upon.

Third, is the type of situation where there is some controversy whether a surgical operation should be done or not, as for example, coronary by-pass surgery for angina pectoris. In case of controversy about surgery, the important thing to keep in mind is, whether the patient would not be worse after it, in so far as looking after himself independently.

Emergency surgery in older people carries a far greater mortality risk and complications after the operation. This is particularly so if the patient is suffering from heart disease, diabetes and liver disorders.

Risk Factors Management.   If the surgical operation is not an emergency, the risk factor present in a particular patient can be assessed and steps taken to minimize their significance. Careful preparation leads to safer surgery. An old person's physiological reserves are diminished and the stress of operation tests him to full. Surgery is often complicated by failure in a system other than that in which the surgeon is operating and in the majority of elderly patients, there are also medical problems which demand consideration.

(a) **Cardiovascular.** An old person who has had a recent heart attack (cardiac infarction), should, if possible, have his operation postponed for three months. A patient with ischemic changes as seen in his ECG, runs a risk of further coronary trouble after surgery. The cerebral circulation also requires consideration. If there is evidence of cerebrovascular insufficiency, operations may be avoided if possible, as there is some risk of stroke. The veins too are important. Thrombophlebitis and pulmonary embolism are among the common complications of surgery. A history of previous thrombophlebitis may give a warning.

(b) **Respiratory.** The greatest hazard of all after surgery is bronchopneumonia. Many old people have bronchitis and a period or treatment with an antibiotic combined with breathing exercises and postural drainage can be of great value. The surgical risk is much reduced if the patient gives up smoking. Attention must be given also to the hygiene of the mouth. Any carious dental stump should be removed. This reduces the risk that the patient with inhale infected material after operation. Common pulmonary complications such as of respiratory insufficiency, pneumonia, lung collapse, occur more often in patients with pre-existing chronic lung disease.

(c) **Kidneys and Bladder.** Operation should be avoided until renal failure has been corrected. The patient should be asked about his bladder function, as incontinence following surgery is common. In men, prostate is examined as retention or urine is a well known complication after any operation.

(d) **Bowels.** Old people are prone to constipation and facial impaction is common. No patient should go to the operation theatre with a loaded rectum.

(e) **Diabetes.** The older patient with diabetes will do better if carefully stabilized before surgery.

(f) **Drugs.** Certain drugs have to be increased before the operation, e.g, corticosteroids.

(g) **Psychological.** The surgeon needs to assess the patient's personality and morale. Anything which can allay his anxiety and depression will be of help.

(h) **Mobility.** Immobility predisposes to pressure sores, so steps need to be taken to make the patient walk as soon as possible.

(i) **Nutrition.** Obese people are more liable to the complications of surgery. If there is time for the patient to lose some weight, he/she may do so. If there is severe anemia, a blood transfusion would be necessary.

(j) **Cardiac Surgery.** It remains an area of controversy. Even though cardiac surgery carries a greater risk for the elderly, the risk/potential benefit relation must be carefully evaluated in order to make the therapeutic choice. Age should never be used as the sole determinant or surgical risk. Other factors, such as general medical condition and presence or absence of pre-existing severe cardiac disease, must be considered. Each case must be individualized. Coronary artery by-pass surgery continues to remain an area of controversy. Recent data suggest that although the preoperative cardiac complication rate (5–10%) is higher in the elderly, continued medical management of left main or three-vessel coronary artery disease may result in an even higher mortality rate.

(k) **Making Anaesthesia Safer.** All anesthetic drugs depress cellular function to a greater or lesser extent. Suitable combination of them and techniques has to be chosen to limit unwanted depression of cellular function, particularly in brain, heart, liver and kidneys. These considerations assume special importance when the surgery is stressful or associated with significant blood loss or tissue trauma.

Preventive Health Care

Prevention of disease is better proposition than cure in any age group. It is much more so in the elderly, because while children and adults may easily recover from a disease, the older persons do so tardily and sometimes only partially. Hence prevention of disease in them carries a much greater significance. Care about prevention of disease in the older patients can be taken at three different stages:

(a) **Primary,** i.e, to prevent illness from taking root and to maintain optimal health.

(b) **Secondary,** i.e, to detect disease at early stages, and to cure it as soon as possible, and

(c) **Tertiary,** to prevent further progression and complication of the disease.

Primary Prevention

This means taking care about the do's and don'ts about health so that the person maintains good health and does not fall ill. The following measures are important in this regard:-

(a) **Adequate Nutritional Intake.** In general, a protein intake of 0.8 gm/kg body weight is sufficient to maintain a positive nitrogen balance. Failure to do so increases risk of infection and fatty infiltration of the liver, etc. Intake of refined glucose should be limited. These foods are low in vitamin and fiber content, and increase risk of dental caries. Carbohydrates should comprise 50 to 60 per cent of most diets. Saturated to unsaturated fat ratio should approximate 1:3 and total fat intake should be limited to not more than 20 percent of calories.

A well balanced diet consisting of at least 1500 to 2000 calories should provide under most circumstances an adequate intake of vitamins and minerals. Although sodium (Salt) intake should be minimized, recent data suggest that only a minority of elderly are "salt-sensitive". In general, sodium intake should not exceed 5 gm/day. Elderly persons rarely require supplemented iron. 1200 to 1500 mg of elemental calcium is the daily recommended requirement. Since many elderly people do not consume a diet high enough in calcium, oral supplementation may be necessary. A well balanced diet should contain the required 15 mg of zinc which has been shown to be essential to wound healing. Sources of dietary zinc include meat, chicken and fish. Adequate fluid intake is essential to maintain normal renal and bowel function. Adequate fiber helps guard against constipation and piles. Fiber must be introduced in the diet slowly so as to avoid intestinal symptoms and poor compliance.

(b) **Avoid increase in weight.** With increasing age, the weight should decrease rather than increase. A weight more than 10 percent of the prescribed height and age table, is a health hazard. Over-weight predisposes to osteoarthritis, diabetes and hypertension and makes a person accident-prone.

(c) **Stop Smoking.** Smoking increases the risk of getting chronic bronchitis and chronic airway obstruction. It increases the risk of getting lung cancer. More frequent upper respiratory tract infections occur in the smokers. Smoking also increases the risk of getting coronary artery disease and the heart attacks. Hence smoking should be stopped.

(d) **Avoid Alcohol.** Changes in body composition that occur with age result in decreased extra and intro cellular fluid compartments. The same intake of alcohol in the elderly as during youth, may now result in a higher effective alcohol level increasing the risk of falls, depression and mental disturbances. The onset of alcoholism is a major problem in the elderly, particularly in men who have recently lost their spouses. Hence alcohol should be avoided.

(e) **Physical Exercise.** Physical exercise is capable of retarding loss of bone mass, improving cardio-pulmonary function, improving mobility and benefiting the psychological profile. Exercise programmes should include isotonic exercises wherein the tone of the muscles remains the same as for example jogging. These consist of full muscles movement without resistance. This is in contrast to isometric exercises wherein the muscle length remains the same. As for example, weight lifting. In the latter, the muscles work against force. These result in excessive increase in peripheral vascular resistance and raised blood pressure. Isometric exercises are not recommended and should be avoided. Exercise should begin gradually and increased slowly.

(f) **Psycho-social Needs.** A comprehensive preventive health care programme must ensure that all psycho-social needs are met. Financial security is necessary to insure adequate nutrition, shelter and medical care. A social network including family, friends and colleagues is essential to optimal functioning. A safe, barrier-free environment should be established. Environmental hazards can include loose rugs, inadequate lighting, stairs and inappropriately placed electric cords and appliances.

(g) **Periodic Health Evaluation.** A yearly comprehensive medical evaluation is recommended for all healthy persons over the age of 60 years. The evaluation should include a thorough history and physical examination.

Secondary Prevention. In order to detect disease tendency to catch disease and to take measures to cure it a thorough physical and laboratory check up is necessary every year after 50 years of age. A check up by cardiologist every year along with lab tests is recommended.

Tertiary Prevention. This involves preventing progression of the disease and its complications. This applies to most of the chronic diseases from which the older people suffer, such as hypertension, diabetes, kidneys, lungs, liver and nervous system disorders etc.

Preventive Hints

Hints to Avoid Constipation

(a) There is no 'normal' number of times one should expect to have a bowel movement each day.

(b) Stay active. Regular exercised increases bowel mobility.

(c) Drink plenty of liquids up six to eight glasses per day, unless you have heart, circulatory or kidney problems. In that case, discuss fluid intake with your physician.

(d) Do not neglect the 'urge' to defecate.

(e) Try emptying your bowels at a preset time each day.

(f) Take advantage of the normal 'gastro colic reflex'; try emptying your bowels 10 to 20 minutes after a hot drink, breakfast or dinner.

(g) Allow adequate time for bowel movements.

(h) Food containing fibers (15 to 30 gm/day) improve bowel function.

(i) Try eating fewer highly processes food such as sweets and fewer foods that are high in fat.

(j) Avoid use of laxatives and/or enemas.

(k) If bowel movements continue to be a problem, see your physician.

Hints to Improve Your Memory.

(a) Be alert and aware. Anything you wish to remember, you must first observe carefully. When you really pay attention, you will become aware of things that ordinarily might make only a vague impression. Since concentration is essential to improving memory, make sure that you are concentrating on one thing at a time and that all forms of distraction are minimized.

(b) Link ideas to images. All memory is based on associating new information to something that you already know. In improving memory, the trick is to link what you want to remember to a strong visual image.

(c) Cure absent-mindedness. Forgetting to turn the gas off or misplacing a set of keys is basically a memory problem. The cure is the trick of association. A timer can help remind you when to turn the gas off, and associating important items, such as keys with specific places in the home can be helpful, for example, you might hang keys on the door knob. Thus you always associated the door knob with your keys.

(d) Be orderly. Forming good habits around the home can help to counteract memory lapses. Medications or dentures should always be kept in the same place. Making lists of things to remember is helpful, as are calendars for remembering birthdays and anniversaries.

(e) Repeat three times. Studies have shown that the most people a new piece of information must be repeated at least three times before it becomes fixed in the memory bank. Some people need as many as 16 repetitions, irrespective of the age. For an even stronger impression of the memory, the idea should be repeated verbally and linked to some visual image.

(f) Organize new information. New information can be remembered more easily if it is organized into categories. Either a mental or written outline can serve as a memory cue. A speech or a lesson can always be remembered more easily if it is arranged in a logical order with particular subheading. Organization can also involve words that help you remember.

(g) Relax and take your time. Memory functions best when you are relaxed and can concentrate. When you are tense, tired or emotionally upset, you cannot expect optimal memory function. Older people cannot absorb too much new information at one time and they may take more time to do so than a younger person. For them, learning just a little at a time may be helpful. If you are unable to recall relatively unimportant information, you should try to avoid anxiety. If you take your mind off it, it very likely will come to you at a later time.

Hints about Avoiding Accidents at Home.

(a) Illuminate all stairways and provide light switches at both top and bottom.

(b) Provide night lights or bedside light switches.

(c) Stairs should preferably have handrails and at a proper height.

(d) Carpets must be tacked down, polished or marble floor should be avoided.

(c) Furniture and other objects must be arranged so that they do not obstruct frequently used walking space.

(f) Non-skid mats or strips should be used in the bath room.

(g) Outdoor steps and walkways must be well lighted and in good repair.

(h) Never smoke in bed or when tired.

(i) When in the kitchen, do not wear flammable synthetic, clothing.

(j) An emergency exit route should be planned and well understood by all household members.

(k) Locks should be secure yet easy to open in times of emergency.

(l) Keep emergency telephones numbers readily accessible.

(m) Use step stools only according to specification and only if someone is present in the house.

(n) Do not climb on ladders, tables or chairs.

(o) Keep off wet floors. Shoes must be well secured and low healed.

(p) Long clothing may also result in falls.

Hints to Make Your Kitchen a Safer Place

(a) Place all shelves at eye level or put commonly used food on the counter. Items in the refrigerator should be stored within easy access.

(b) Avoid excessive bending or reaching out for something. Use of chair and ladders can be dangerous. Step stools must be sturdy.

(c) All chairs should have heavy backs, arm, rests, and non-slip legs. The seat should be of appropriate height to allow easy ability to get on and off the chair.

(d) Clean up spills promptly.

(e) Use slippers with non-skid soles.

(f) Have adequate lighting in the kitchen, especially around cooking and cutting areas.

(g) Do not wear long or loose clothing in the kitchen. Clothing should be made of non-inflammable materials. Plastic aprons can be hazardous.

(h) Store all appliances, utensils, and cooking accessories in secured and marked areas.

(i) A light weight fire extinguisher should be within easy reach.

(j) Have emergency telephone numbers pasted near the kitchen telephone.

Important Hints For Food

Food

1. Do not try to bite or break hard objects with your teeth. Your teeth may break.

2. Try to eliminate deep-fried things from your food.

3. Take at least ½ litre of milk daily.

4. Take a little less quantity of diet than your stomach demands or your tongue relishes. Do not over-eat.

5. You should supplement your diet with a tablet of multivitamins and minerals.

6. Avoid alcohol.

7. Stop smoking, if you are a smoker.

Physical Exercise

1. Take morning walk daily. Do not run after 60 years of age. Jog on green grass for 15 minutes.

2. Physical exercise or Yoga exercises must be done daily. If you don't do so as yet, start slowly and gradually.

Taking Medicines

1. Long years of taking medicines for various ailments have not made you an expert in the field. Take the advice of the doctor, if you do not feel well.

2. Throw away the long-kept medicines in your cupboard or drawers.

3. Remember, youth cannot be brought back. Use of excitatory drugs, stimulants, hormones or aphrodisiacs increases the wear and tear of the body.

4. Avoid colouring your hair with any chemical solution, if it causes irritation in your scalp.

5. Avoid use of sleeping pills as far as possible.

Avoiding Accidents

1. Cross the road very carefully. Your strength and your reflexes are weak now, and they may leave you in lurch in the middle of the road.

2. Walk carefully. Scan the ground for any depression, pits or obstructions.

3. Better avoid climbing the ladders or high stools.

Reduce Obesity

1. Obesity increases chances of getting accidents.

2. Obesity increases chances of suffering from:-

   (a) Diabetes.

   (b) Hypertension.

   (c) Arthritis.

3. Obesity reduces the life-span. So try to bring back your weight to normal or within plus/ minus 10 percent or your age.

Consulting Your Doctor

1. If you do not feel well, see your doctor and follow his advice.

2. Get your teeth and gums checked up and property conditioned at least once a year.

3. Get your vision tested, if you have difficulty in reading.

4. Get yourself physically checked up yearly.

5. If your doctor advises, get your blood tested for hemoglobin, urine for routine examination including albumin and sugar and ECG if indicated.

6. Women above forty should get Pap-Cervical smear test done yearly.

7. Women above forty should learn to examine their breasts fortnightly according to instructions set out by the family doctor.

Plan Your Day

1. Plan your day for better utilization of time.

2. Plan your week, month and year. Plan the next decade as to what you intend to achieve.

3. Try not to fritter away your time and energy in only day-to-day work.

4. Try to reduce unnecessary speech, thought and action. Learn to sit in meditation.

5. Think how you wish to be remembered after death and what you have to do now in this regard.

6. Try more to give, rather than to get.

Chapter-3

Wealth the Second Happiness

(Money makes the mare go)

A proverb

Financial Security

Sound financial state is the second most important factor after health to make our life happy and comfortable. There goes a popular saying, "Money makes the mare go". I would like to convert this into a practical saying that "Financial security makes the retired and old horse to canter". To be young and not be financially sound is normal and can be tolerated but to be old and retired and not be financially sound can be disastrous. Though, it is generally said that "money is not everything in life" but what I say is that it not everything but it is something which, if you do not have, when you really need it, it can be a very sorrowful and miserable state.

The generation born after our adulthood i.e, born after 1970 is quite aware of the importance of being financially sound. In fact, they are two steps ahead of our generation in this field. Our generation, born between 1947–1969 i.e, post independent generation is quite clueless about personal financial management. I remember some of our seniors and colleagues used to face problems in paying their monthly officers mess bill. Today it is not so and our youngsters are well aware and it is worth learning from them.

Saving and Investment

The purpose of savings and investments while in service and after retirement are three folds:-

- Have reasonable carry home salary/pension/income for normal living during service and even after retirement.
- Have maximum tax benefits by saving. These savings should augment your income after retirement.
- Investments should give reasonable returns, be risk free and fairly liquid to draw.

Options

One should not save too much for the future to feel uncomfortable while in service and as such there is no guarantee that you may live to enjoy these savings. Therefore, save wisely for your post retirement days. Some of the factors which can help you in selecting various saving options available are:-

- Safety of the savings.
- Amount of returns.
- Liquidity.
- Tax benefits.
- Your risk taking profile.

If you consider various options in the field of investment then these could be:-

- Provident Fund including Public Provident Fund.
- Fixed deposits with banks and post offices.
- Real estate investments.
- Equity or equity related mutual funds.
- Debt related funds of bonds.

In order to find out what suits you best the following decision matrix should be of help considering that your risk taking profile is good:-

Factors / Saving Options	Safety	Returns	Tax Benefit	Liquidity	Risk Profile of Investor	Total
PPF (PF)	5	3	3	4	2	17
FDs	3	1	2	5	1	12
Real Estate	4	5	1	3	4	17
Equity	2	4	1	2	5	16
Bonds	1	2	1	1	3	9

The table above is for a high risk profile investor as he has graded 5 and 4 opposite real estate and equity related investments under returns. The grading has been done with best preference being graded 5 and lowest being as 1. In the above matrix the priority of investment should be as under:-

P1 - PPF (14)

P2 - Real Estate (17)

P2 - Equity (16)

P3 - FDs (12)

P4 - Bonds (10)

Priority options for this investor.

In the table above, all factors are equally weighted and their grading is allotted by a particular risk taker as per his preferences. There is yet another method of preparing the matrix i.e., grading the factors. In this method you grade the factors as per your preference. One example is:-

Factor		Grading
Safety	-	**16**
Returns	-	**12**
Tax benefits	-	**8**
Liquidity	-	**4**

Now prepare the table and find out the solutions as per your risk profile and preferences as under:-

Factors / Saving Options	Safety	Returns	Tax Benefit	Liquidity	Total
PPF (PF)	16	8	8	2	34
FDs	12	4	2	4	22
Real Estate	8	12	0	3	23
Equity	0	10	6	1	19
Bonds	4	6	4	0	10

With this matrix PPF (PF) remains top priority sector and Real Estate comes second priority sector. It will be seen from above analysis that priority saving sectors for a salaried person PF/PPF. As you should not put all your eggs in one basket, you should now decide on percentage in first three investments. Savings in PPF/PF are generally best options for all serving personnel and contribution should be made to get maximum tax benefits.

Investment in Housing or Real Estate

One of the primary and necessary requirements for a person is to have his own roof over his head. With the boost to housing sector and benefits available to the investor, this is one of the best investments today. Some of the factors which should be considered before taking this decision are:-

(a) Place of investment i.e. town or city.

(b) When i.e. at what time in service to invest.

(c) What type of investment i.e. house or plot, agricultural or farm land?

As far as place of investment is concerned this should be around your area of domicile or influence. If you hail from Rajasthan and invest in Bangalore/Trivandrum you may not find it convenient to take care of it and also the disposal, when desired so, becomes difficult. Let us say you are from Jaipur then your investments in real estate should be at Jaipur, Alwar, jodhpur, Gurgaon or New Delhi including Noida. If you come from a floating family then you have to decide on the place after due consideration with near and dear ones. Places around, say 100–150 kms, from a metro have scope for appreciation and future development.

As regards the time of investment, it should be done at such a time that the loan on property should have been completely paid back by the time you decide to retire. If we take 30 years as an average service span then anytime between 8 to 10 years of service is the ideal time for you to invest in this sector. Firstly, you would have got married and you should have some savings in your provident fund. For the next 20 years the house should be kept on rent and keep paying the loan out of the rent. This investment will ensure a roof over your head when you retire, the property would have been paid out by the rent received and you would have enjoyed maximum tax benefits in service. Tax benefits in housing sector are likely to continue for next 20–25 years.

What type of investment should be made is again a deliberate decision? Making or constructing a house by you, while in service, is a big botheration. It is, therefore, recommended that you should buy a house/flat in a place where rental values are good. You should also invest in a plot so that you can make a house before retirement either by disposing off the flat you had purchased while in service or by taking loan again. How big or what kind of house or flat can be purchased depends on your repayment capacity and rental values in that town. Having a roof over your head is a very important factor in giving you financial and social security after retirement. I know of a Major General who retired from service without making a house for him. He had to spend his retired life in a officers institute with one room accommodation in a very embarrassing situation. In order to remain financially happy you should retire without any liability of loans.

Investments- Retirement benefits

When a person retires after 30 to 35 years of service or so he is likely to receive a good amount as retirement benefits with these are in the form of:-

(a) Gratuity

(b) Commutation

(c) AGIF

(d) Provident Fund

(e) Encashment on leave

Let us assume that, on an average, you will have 50 lakhs rupees to invest after retirement. The balance amount out of this will actually depend upon your social obligations too. If your children are settled and married, your house is already constructed and if you have purchased a new car then the whole amount less what is needed by you as reserve can be invested. The factors which should be considered are same as given under normal investment previously. A suggested portfolio for an investment of Rs 50 lacs is as under:-

(a) Rs. 9 Lakhs in monthly income scheme of post office for retired personnel in two names with benefits of section 80L of Income tax Act.

(b) Rs.1.5 Lakhs (Rs one and half lakhs per year in PPF including tax saving bonds.

(c) Rs.20 Lakhs in long term growth related equity related mutual funds. (Invest in only blue chip companies with sound fundamentals).

(d) Rs.20 Lakhs in share market to be kept in short term bank or post office deposits. Post office account with also help in receiving monthly interest from (a) above.

This investment will take care of regular inflow of cash from Ser (a) and (d) which will augment your monthly income. Ser (b) and (c) will take care of long term growth and income for future. Investment in PPF should help you in saving income tax. Here you may be advised that after retirement you may find some of your near and dear ones asking for financial help.

You would have to decide on this issue yourself as **"money is a very dicey object and is capable of souring sweetest of relationships"**.

I would conclude this chapter by highlighting the following:-

(a) Invest maximum in PPF/PF up to 10 to 15 years of service. Thereafter review, if needed.

(b) Retirement benefits must be invested with due care.

(c) Must make use of maximum tax benefits as this helps you as well as state by savings.

(d) Invest in flat or house around 8 to 10 years of service in a town having good rental values.

(e) Invest in a plot for future in which payment can be made by EMI. A farm house of farm land can also be purchased if it can be gainfully exploited after possession.

(f) Finally remember, in most cases, once you retire, your own house and your own saving will come very handy. Your investment plan should be such that your income after retirement is, at least, equal to your carry home salary at the time of retirement.

(g) You must take a mediclaim insurance policy well in time if not covered by your family.

You must remember the good old saying by a psychologist that hard cash in the form of bank balance does give a feeling of happiness but do not forget to save for the remaining life or the rainy day. You should also make a living "Will" to show distribution of your wealth after you and your spouse's death.

Chapter-4

Family & Social Life

(Man is a social animal)

Old saying

If you have been able to look after your health and finances then the next important factor, in order to live happily, is 'Social Security'. It may be slightly difficult to define social security in exact words but it is definitely not abstract. Various elements which constitute social security are:-

- Financial security.
- Family happiness and status.
- Company of colleagues, near and dear ones.
- Individual social status.
- Fulfilling one's domestic and social obligations successfully.
- Desire to live longer in the society.

It can, therefore, be presumed that a person is socially secure if he is financially sound, has a reasonable individual and family status, has reasonable social circuit or company of his own, his social obligations are performed well and he has desire to live in the society. To summerise- "A man should not be social discard and should have desire to live longer in the society". Remember good old sayings- **"Man is a social animal"** and **"No man is an island"**.

You have to plan and execute certain actions to ensure that you are socially happy after your retirement. While in service you have your family, colleagues, subordinates and superiors who keep you occupied. After your retirement, at best if you are lucky, you may have your spouse and some of your likeminded people to give you company. It is said that a man keeps losing everything in life except his wife. Your marriage, therefore, is the most important milestone in your life. Your parents would have left for Godly abode, your children may be employed or staying separately, your service colleagues would have gone but your wife is with you throughout your life, if you are fortunate. You have to get married to a lady who is not only likeminded but also a good companion in old age. I have seen some old couples living together under the same roof but otherwise living in two different worlds. At this stage your social behaviour, your spiritual urges, your eating habits, health and of course, your thinking should be in complete harmony with that of your life partner. You would have got married anytime after 25/26 years of age but well before 29/30 years. This ensures that you have spent good enough life together before you start facing retirement and old age blues. Marriage should take place after a reasonable period of courting and knowing each other well. If you get married well before thirty years of age then in most circumstances, your children would have completed their education and they would have, at least, been professionally settled before you retire. In case you get married late then you have to be mentally prepared to be either doing baby sitting or at least remain worried about your children after your retirement. You should ideally plan in such a way that before you retire you should have completed your obligation of your children's education and settlement in professional careers. In case of a female child (daughter) she must be married off before your retirement.

Social Company

You should not become a "nagging husband" after retirement. We keep talking about nagging wives all over while in service but it should not become the reverse after retirement. You and your spouse should find some social and spiritual company. It can be in the field of sports, cards, and club or bhajan kirtan. As I have mentioned earlier, wine and woman can keep the man desirous of living longer but I would like to reiterate this here that moderate drink, company of our own woman and some kind of music, song and dance can keep anyone willing to live happily and healthy. One must not join a social company of drunkards and gamblers just for the fun of it. I have seen a function in a Senior Living Project which was more like life extending happiness event.

Better Half a Better Company

Retired life is a period when most of your time is going to be spent with your wife. At best you may have a servant around you who has been faithful to you, otherwise the life is going to revolve around you and your better half. Of course, it is not the time and stage of convert her into "My fair lady", but you can definitely make her a better company. The basic formula is harmony and if you translate this magic word into Punjabi and call it "Haar-Manny" (accept her defeat) you will be the best husband and couple in the town. It is actually a necessity of old age to be complementary to each other rather than indifferent.

In order to make her a good companion, if you have not already done so during service, please take the following steps immediately:-

- Take her for a walk daily. She being younger in age (3 to 5 years), will be able to give you a good company.
- Eat together. Adjust to a common menu.
- Go to a social club together.
- Try and teach her some dancing and singing bhajan or song only for you.
- See that she keeps a good health.
- Teach her driving a car.
- Follow the basic dictum of "share and care".

Vices

To be a happy and healthy retired man you should drop all vices, minor as well major. Some of these need to be shunned urgently. For a start you should:-

- Become a vegetarian.
- Consume liquor as medicine. "Sau dawa ek daru"- A Rajasthani saying meaning one peg of brandy is equal to a hundred medicines. Just be, what is called, a 'social drinker'.
- Leave smoking if you are a smoker.
- Interest in one's own spouse must continue. This may not be only for romance but also for each other's good company and for sharing and caring.

Interaction with Children and Relatives

Once you have retired and your children have settled down in their careers and life, frankly speaking, you have no longer a role to play. You have grown, flowered, thrown your seeds and are now actually withering. You have done your bit, and that's it. The only thing we can give to our children is our wisdom which at most times is not needed. A few important Don'ts and Do's to have very happy and healthy relation with your children at this stage of life are given below:-

Don'ts

- Do not give sermons to your children.
- Do not blow your own trumpet.
- Do not give advice if not asked for.
- Do not be a teacher or a butcher.
- Do not interfere in their life and career.
- Do not coach them for upbringing their children.

Do's

- Do help them financially, when needed for asked for.
- Do advise them when asked for.
- Do spend some time with them, at least a fortnight or so in a year.
- Do interact like a grand old man with your grand children.
- Do keep in touch with them, if they are in a different place both by telephones and by writing an occasional note.
- Do help your children during birth of their children.

If you analyse above do's and Don'ts you will find these are nearly same actions in positive and negative forms. Let me emphasis it again- "DO NOT" interfere with them but interact and help as and when asked for.

Social Service

This is an ideal stage to devote some time and help to the society. This could be in the fields of education, health and hygiene, environment protection, poverty alleviation and child development. I know of a retired Lt Gen who, along with his wife, conducts English and Maths classes for children, who are good at studies but can't afford to pay extra tuition. Lt Gen and Mrs Baljeet Singh (a gunner officer) had retired and settled down in an Adivasi belt in Jharkhand State and were running a school for the children. A retired L/Naik of ASC, Anna Hazare has been awarded "Padma Shree' in Maharashtra State for his dedication in the field of forest and environmental protection. Army personnel specially officers who retire from service after 25 to 30 years of service have good amount of administrative capability and fair amount of energy to undertake such pursuits. Your organizational strength, team spirit and experience as a veteran should be put to a proper use in the field or your liking. An Armed Forces officer/JCO is best suited for education management, teaching and general administration.

While in service, we remain away from society and or relatives. We live in a restricted and disciplined circle of our duty. Now, after retirement, you are a free bird with tons and tons of experience, plenty of energy, grand ideas and freedom of action, which should be exploited to the maximum. You must contribute to society whatever you can and whatever extent you can afford.

Finally to conclude this important aspect of social security, I would say that if you have taken care of your health and finances then half of your social security is already in place. Some people are of the opinion that "let the society be damned, as long as I am healthy and I have enough money to buy my requirements". This may be alright for a short period. Now you are not on your annual leave that after two months you will go back to your unit or Headquarters and you have nothing to lose or gain from the society. Here, you have come for good and society definitely expects you to contribute and interact as per your status and organization you have retired from.

Hobbies and Pastime

When you retire from active service, you will find plenty of time at your disposal. Unlike in service where you keep saying, where is the time? At this age you are likely to sleep less, you will have no official or time bound commitments and you may find that you are entering the arena of boredom. With reduced company of near and dear ones, you would definitely need to spend some leisure moments in some useful manner. It is, therefore, most important that you develop a hobby before retirement. Your hobbies could be:-

- Gardening.
- Playing some musical instrument.
- Taking long walks.
- Golf.
- Swimming.
- Freelance writing.
- Joining a Bhajan- Kirtan group.

- Joining a health club.
- Playing cards.
- Bird watching.
- Cleanliness is next to Godliness.

A hobby is, basically, an activity which you like to undertake to spend your spare time and which you like to do from the core of your heart to give you satisfaction. While selecting a hobby, in addition to liking it from within, you should ensure that it is affordable as well as easily available in the station. If you decide to retire and stay in your farm house then you may not be able to play golf every day. But if you think golf or swimming is a passion with you and you are staying at your village or farm house then you should find some time, say once a week or once a month, to go and play golf or swim somewhere in a nearby town where these facilities exist. Hence, you may like to become an out station member of these clubs. A hobby provides great satisfaction to your mind and soul and keeps your heart and mind young. Hence the importance of hobby or passion to be fulfilled.

As I have stated earlier that you will find plenty of time to yourself after retirement, this time should be utilized to do something constructive. And a set routine should also be followed to avoid boredom and to keep yourself physically and mentally occupied. On week days a suggested time chart for a retired person can be as under:-

Time Chart

	Summer	Winter
	(Apr – Oct)	(Nov – Mar)
• Rise in the morning	0500 Hours	0600 Hours
• Morning walk	0530–0630	0700–0800

	Summer	**Winter**
• Yoga/aerobics/Exercise	0630–0700	0800–0830
• Bath, Breakfast etc	0700–0800	0830–0930
• Reading newspaper, Magazine, TV etc.	0800–0900	0930–1000
• Hobby - Indoor/Social Service	0900–1200	1000–1200
• Helping hand to your Wife	1200–1230	1200–1330
• Lunch	1300–1400	1330–1400
• Rest (Reading, Watching TV and Siesta for not more Than half an hour)	1400–1700	1400–1600
• Hobby (outdoor) or Social Service	1700–1900	1600–1700
• Evening with family	1900–2200	1700–2200
• Sleep	2200–0500	2200–0600

This table is not a time table for a trainer or a person under training that it should be followed as given. But it is very important to follow a routine so that your body and mind remain active. As long as you have spent seven hours for sleep, two hours for physical activity, five to six hours for hobby or social work and remaining nine to ten hours with your wife and family, you have followed a reasonably active time chart for a retired person. On weekends you must plan a small outdoor activity and this could be in the form of a small hike, going around the golf course or as a small picnic or outing. The most important thing to remember is to break the daily monotony which is responsible for boredom. On some occasions/ weekends you can visit your relatives, parents and other friends who are living away from you. Having retired from your job you should not retire from life. You have to ensure that:-

- You do not become a nagging husband.

- You remain physically and mentally active.

- You don't allow lethargy to set in, and therefore follow a reasonably active routine as suggested.

- Let boredom not be allowed to overtake you and make you feel lethargic or overpowered.

- Let your passion and hobby be exploited for physical and psychological satisfaction.

- Let there be some interest in music, song and dance so that the desire of living a wholesome life is kept alive.

- Let you not be trapped in the company of gamblers, card players and drug addicts who will make you a "sitting duck" rather than a cantering horse.

Chapter-5

Retirement – A Hard Fact of Life

(Retire you will, crib you may, but remember the life can re-start at sixty again)

A happy view.

Retirement from one's job, service, business or work is sure shot event which has to take place one or the other day. Does this retirement from one's job, work, business or service mean retirement from life, pleasures of life, happiness of life and social and moral responsibilities and obligations? I suppose, and you will agree with me, that it does not! Retirement simply means retirement from one's job/service/business. All your responsibilities and obligations stand as they are at the point in time.

I am quite sure that you will not stop enjoying life just because you have retired from your job. In fact, only your obligation of office timing, your obligation to your boss and subordinates and your official engagements will cease and you are likely to find time for yourself, your family and your friends whom, so far, you were not able to find due to your job/work/ business or service. In order to devote this available time, you will now have to find something to do, which is precisely the aim of this book.

You have to prepare yourself for this important event. Your income is likely to go down and you will have your social and moral obligations at hand. You will have plenty of time but you will have to find ways and means to usefully utilize the same. You would have crossed over to wrong side of sixty and hence be more careful about your health.

While preparing for retirement you will have to consider quite a few issues in details like where to settle down after retirement? What job/work to find? How to keep yourself busy, healthy, wealthy and happy? I remember when one of our family friends was to retire in 1999; she wrote a very sentimental letter which made me read that letter time and again. My retirement, at that time, was still some six years away. Sentiments which she had expressed about how her family had spread all over, how she was left all alone and how she is preparing herself to work for the "Santhome Church" in Chennai after retirement made me read that letter three to four times. I had, really, not realized the hard facts of retirement which in my case were still a little away. However, based on her letter and sentiments I started my preparations and decided to make a house for myself.

One of the Generals of Post independent India Lt General ML Chibber who was awarded Padam Bhushan for his services once described the formula of satisfaction/happiness which states:-

$$\text{Satisfaction \% } = 1/\alpha \, \frac{\text{Number of desires desired}}{\text{Number of desires fulfilled}}$$

For example, if you desire to own a Mercedes Car and in due course of time you have it then you are fully satisfied. But if you had desired to own a Mercedes Car, a flat in Mumbai/Goa, a farm house in Jaipur and a summer resort in Almora and in due course of time you only own a Mercedes Car then your satisfaction level is 25% only. This, of course is a philosophical approach. If you can control your desires then you are going to be a Sadhu/Sanyasi!! Is it also practical? First you want or desire a Mercedes Car and then restrain your desire and say I can also be happy or satisfied with a Wagon-R!!!

Satisfaction is also synonymous with Happiness, Enjoyment, pleasure, easement, fulfillment, success, Gladness, Content, Blessed and a few other words which are used by people like cloud Nine, on top of the world etc etc. This book is basically meant to describe the state of satisfaction of a person form personal, family, societal and spiritual point of view. The scope looks too wide but it has been simplified for a normal human being. I would personally describe the state of happiness as follows:-

Desire/Aim/Mission/Target/Objective

⇩

Planned & Execution.

⇩

Achievement/Fulfillment

⇩

Happiness

⇩

Satisfaction

While you are in a job/service, you generally remain occupied physically and mentally and you have little time to complain. After retirement, you have all the time in the world and if you are not happy or satisfied then you will make your life miserable. Some ideas to remain happy, healthy, occupied and satisfied are suggested after 15 years of satisfied and experience of retirement.

Retirement from service is a hard fact like death after birth. Everyone has to retire from service one day or the other. Many of us do realize the hard fact that we have to retire one day but we tend to ignore the harsh facts of retirement. The changes in life style, withdrawal of service perks of the rank or appointment while in the service and more materially the reduced income; really bring in what is called "post retirement blues'. The state is something very close to midlife blues, when you are struggling with life. In mid life you have growing family, rising expenditures, future of your own career, children education, wife's health and career and frequent transfers of posting are some of the problems of mid life. Then, lack of company, reduced income, old age and deteriorating health of self and spouse and finally in some cases, regret and remorse are some of post retirement problems.

"If I had _ _ _ _ _ _ _" or "I wish I could _ _ _ _ _ _ _ _ _ " are some of the regrettable words or sentences which people often talk after retirement. In fact one must analyse the hard and harsh facts of post retirement life and prepare himself to overcome these as part of the preparation for retirement.

Hard Facts

Some hard facts about retirement are:-

- You will retire on so and so date.
- You will need a house to live in.
- Your income will reduce to nearly half after retirement.

- Service perks will stand withdrawn.
- You will need a suitable conveyance.

Harsh Facts

Some harsh facts are:-

- You may not have the company of colleagues, children or family.
- Your health may deteriorate due to age or sickness.
- You will need to maintain a reasonable status as per your last rank or appointment held in service.
- Your chances of earning more may continue to reduce as you grow older and older.
- Regret and remorse may not help you.

Acclimatization

The word acclimatization is used in high altitude areas and it is a process of getting used to that altitude and environment. Once you get posted to a high altitude area from plains you suddenly find yourself in an uncomfortable environment due to lack of oxygen and extreme cold climate. Similarly, one has to acclimatize to the fact of retirement and be prepared to get used to harsh facts of a retired life. Like the process of acclimatization for a period of seven days, one has to work for six to seven years before you actually retire. This period can be utilized for creating an environment and working conditions for you to settle down in post retirement life. Activities which you have to complete well before retirement are:-

- Have a roof over your head ie; make a house for yourself in a town where the cost of living suits your post retirement life. A town close to, say 100 to 150 KM, away from metro may provide you such an opportunity.

- Buy a new conveyance (Car/Jeep/Motor Cycle/ Scooter) depending upon your requirement and affordability before you retire. This will serve your for 10-15 years after your retirement and save you a lot of time, money and inconvenience of spending time with a mechanic in a garage.

- Develop a hobby as a pastime. It could be golf, swimming, freelance writing, gardening, social work or joining a bhajan mandali for spiritual upliftment.

- Investments before and after retirement should be made in such a way that these supplement your reduced income in a reasonable manner i.e.; at least equal to the last carry home pay.

- Develop an attitude of:-
  - Generosity and forgiveness.
  - Detachment from family especially children.
  - Be a good listener and silent observer.
  - Avoid moral lectures to your near and dear ones.
  - Serving the humanity or society if you are left with some strength.

In fact what is needed for a retired life is:-

- Peace and harmony.
- Good health.
- Financial security.

- Social security.
- Affordable hobby.
- And of course, God's grace and blessings.

I have tried to include most of what is needed after retirement in this book. I have also included some actions or activities to be undertaken at various stages of life to overcome the problems after retirement and draw maximum benefits out of these activities during service. Remember, retirement is not just an event in your career but an important milestone which requires advances planning, thinking and taking a number of actions well before you actually retire. The details of various activities are given in succeeding chapters. The details will include as to when making a house, how much and what type of investments should you indulge in while in service, how should you invest your post retirement benefits etc. These forthcoming chapters will also include as to what should be your concern as far as your health is concerned and what kind of social and psychological attitude you should build before retirement.

Retirement from service or job does not mean retirement form life. You must remember that life actually begins at 60 when you are the boss of yourself. So far, you were serving your boss and now you are the boss.

Chapter-6

Happiness and Circus of Life

(Happiness is tonic of life)

Advice.

Ghalib had sad, "I have got some clues about heaven", but don't you think it's only a good idea to console yourself? Some people say that if there is heaven, it is here on this earth and if there is hell then also it is here on the earth. Well even if you feel there is a heaven and a hell 'up above' then why don't you work towards going to that heaven? Why do we go for each other's throat? Why are we divided so much on petty issues? Even in the twenty first century – we are fighting on issues on which animal, too, have stopped fighting! Let us leave this heaven and hell issue for some time and see how we can make residual life worth living. If you are not happy after retirement, you alone are to be blamed. When we were born, the average life expectancy was 28 years. We have outlived twice that limit and we are not on God's great bonus. Let us enjoy and celebrate the fact of being alive. Therefore, enjoy every moment and live it up and kick it up!

Be Yourself

The easiest thing in the world is to be yourself. The best way of living happily is to be your own self with complete originality in you. There is that Shakespearean concept of this world being a stage and every man and woman being an actor. Well that may be alright when you were on the stage i.e, while you were in service, you had your subordinates, superiors and peers to act with. After retirement you are on the stage of being all by yourself. Therefore, be yourself and be happy. You do not have to copy any one, compete with anyone or outshine anybody around you.

Laughter, the Best Medicine

Even if God has not been kind in that he has not given you that natural sense of good humour then you can definitely make an effort to develop it now. Join a laughing club if you do not feel that you can laugh on your own. In this field I would advise you to develop the attitude of Sikh community to laugh on yourself first. If you can laugh at yourself then you have an excuse as well as right to laugh at others. I would like to draw your attention to the following few lines on "Sense of Humour":-

Sense of Homour

What makes you laugh,

And saves you from cough.

Can keep you away from TB and tumour,

It's nothing but good sense of humour.

Among living species only human have,

Other senses even birds and animals have.

A little smile on your face,

Can add enough charm and grace.

'Laughter, the best medicine' can keep the doc away,

God's given humour can keep you on the sway.

Learn to laugh on yourself first,

As laughing on others is not just.

Sarcasm adds disease to humour,

Gossip can turn it into a rumour.

Impersonal, simple and lighter side,

Can keep the humour neat and tide.

Crib you may but laugh you must,

But remember to laugh at yourself first.

Remember, when you were young and you thought you could knock the mountain down, cloud the sun and what not! But if you remember well then you would realize that actually you could not do much. Now that you are old and retired, you do not have a captive audience of your subordinates to laugh on your dry sense of humour or Pjs (poor Jokes), your superiors on whose jokes you could laugh at, you should, therefore, learn to laugh at yourself. Laugh aloud and merrily and do not put any artificial accent to it. Remember you can't alter the height of Mount Everest, you can't change the course of The Ganges or The Yamuna, you can't change the direction of the blowing wind, but you can definitely laugh and laugh as much you can. Laughter is not only useful for feeling better; it also helps in good blood circulation. Most people with good sense of humour generally live longer and keep a youngish profile.

I know about a General who was my Corps Commander. He was six years older than and senior by eight years to me in service. But his sense of humour was twenty five years younger than mine. This was one of the factors that the General kept his disposition twenty five years younger. Hence, smile as it adds grace to your face. Live it up and be happy.

Some Important Tips

In addition to "being yourself" and "laughing at yourself" some important tips to feel happy and young are:-

- Spend some time with your children and grand children. They say that young company has a 'rub off' effect on you and it makes you feel happy and young. You may like to behave like a typical grand old man telling stories of old times or listen to children's stories, songs or jokes. Also play children's games and watch children's films. These children may not be of your own family. Remember, child is the father of man and old people are more like children in many respects.

- Develop some interest in dance and music. Every one may not be able to sing well or dance well but you can definitely watch others dance and listen to their songs. It is a researched fact that in addition to **wine and woman, music and dance** also make you feel happy and healthy.

- Do not be a habitual watcher of horror or late night movies. In fact you should watch some children movies, cartoon films and gentle moderate sex comedy or serial films. These provide you enough stimulation and humour.

- Last but not the least, do not try and become a fault finder for your own family and for the society. For God's sake and in the interest of your own health, please do not start thinking at this stage, that every bloody thing is wrong in this world.

- Do "aish" till you really become ash or earth?

Never Envy Others Happiness

One of the best ways to be happy is to share others happiness. Like we share grief of family, friends and peers we should also share happiness of others. It is commonly believed that most people are sad and unhappy due to success, happiness and joy of others. Even animals don't do that. Never envy others for their happiness.

The Circus of Life

William Shakespeare had described the world as a stage and life as a play or drama in his famous Play "As you like it". As men and women, we play our roles and fade away. After more than five hundred years, there are great differences in social environment and role we live and play in twenty first century. Life has become a full fledged circus and we try to live it as an infant, child, teenager, adult, parents and finally we get senile and depart from here for the next journey. Meera Nair, a modern film producer, had once remarked, "I love circus of life and love layering it". How correct and perfect she is? Both Shakespeare and Meera Nair have inspired me to write these limericks of life. We all try to live and layer our lives. There is an old saying that after crossing sixty years of age, we generally say that one has gone senile. Today life, starts at sixty when we retire. In my first book titled "Retire rich Happy and Healthy" which I had compiled three years after my retirement, I had written that retirement is as important a phase of life as pre-retirement. The observations and advice in this booklet are totally related to present day scenario.

I have based writing of this booklet on my observations through seventy years of age and having seen through four generations in my little world.

1. The Circus of Life

The life is creation of God and nature,
At different stages we act different creature.

At birth we bring the greatest pleasure,
This moment is beyond any measure.

As an infant, you are wonderful source of joy,
As a child in the lap, you are a playful toy.

Up to ten or so, you are fairly ignorant,
But as teenager you become quite arrogant.

Adulthood brings some pains and gains,
You try to hold your horses¹ by reigns.

Mid life² blues make you black and blue,
Wife, family, career and you have no clue.

Mid life becomes the most crucial stage,
Because this lasts up to fifty years of age.

Maturity and parenting at crucial fifty,
Makes you conceit, confused and thrifty.

---

¹Mind games
²Remaining life.

Then you are on other side of the hill,
You are left with residual years and the ills.

Suddenly the retirement knocks at your door,
You are left with your savings and no more.

Retirement is yet a little difficult phase,
With loneliness, weakness and advanced age.

You try to serve the purpose of life and detach,
But you remain confused and you can't catch.[3]

Most pleasures of life turn into pains,
With old age you can't see the gains.

Your actions[4] *pay you here and right,*
With pains and spasm you begin to fight.

The final act is eternal and full peace,
If you have toiled for such a treatise.

---

[3]Can't understand.
[4]Karma.

2. Birth the Beginning

Your birth is outcome of love and need,
For sake of gen next and biological greed.

Your arrival is welcome by one and all,
Near and dear merrily celebrate tall.

The mid wife cleans and cuts,
Your umbilical cord and all the nuts.[5]

Then you are wrapped softly with utter care,
Every one waits for you to cry and snare.

Then they anxiously and curiously wait,
For you to defecate and urinate.

Some say you look like Mom,
Other say you look like Tom.[6]

Your Mom clings to you like dove,
Grandparents simply and tenderly love.

You become Papa's bundle of joy,
For rest of the family a beautiful toy.

---

[5]Unwanted folds in the cord.
[6]Father

Grandparents glare at you with pride,
Others enjoy the pleasant sight and stride.
The family throws a treat for all,
Near and dear perceive very tall.[7]

In some places if born as a boy,
You bring endless pleasure and joy.

But if born as a girl in some places,
The family develops unpleasant traces.

---

[7]Proud

3. The Infancy

From birth to two years of age,
You are cumbersome to manage.

Infancy is absolute delicate norm,
Both for family and your mom.

You are loved with care,
No one can neglect and dare.[8]

Your sight itself gives pleasure.
And treated like hidden treasure,

You are protected and cared like honey,
Also cared and loved better than money.

Infancy ends when you start walking,
Especially when you start yapping.

---

[8]Threaten, Challenge

4. *The Childhood*

Your childhood begins with a bang,
You are made to join the school gang.

You are forced to go to Pre School,
You too, play tricks like a fool.

A donkey's load on your back,
May be you are lighter than that sack.

Your gait shows utter complexity,
Your reluctance ignored with anxiety.

You are pushed into the school van,
While you try to turn turtle and tan.

You start getting work for home,
You don't bother who does it at home.

Home work becomes worst past time,
Though, mom does it most of the time.

At times there comes a feeling,
Your childhood, someone is stealing.

Your childhood and all the pleasure,
Simply stolen without any measure.

Then school becomes second home,
With Ena, Joe, Piki, and Tom.[9]

After a while you become chatterbox,
No one listens but you shout like a fox.

Friends, friends and friends galore,
Play more and more, with little snore.

Childhood becomes a real pleasure,
With friends becoming a hidden treasure.

---

[9]School friends

5. Adolescence and Teenage

When friendship circle suddenly increases,
And interest in books and studies decreases.

You like to go out and simply play,
Among friends and friends you like to sway.

When you learn to say 'NO' to everything,
Only friends and friends mean something.

When you are able to simply differentiate,
Between 'boy and girl' then you are on teen's gate.

When you realize that you are someone,
Then you have crossed the age of eleven.

This curious life is called teens,
And you start realizing your beans.

When your body and voice mature,
You at times feel quite insecure.

At thirteen you try to rake up,
At fourteen you try to shake up.

At fifteen you start preaching,
At sixteen you start teaching.

At seventeen romantic feeling set in,
At eighteen the opposite sex is let in.

At nineteen you are knocking at adulthood
You feel why every place is not Holly wood.

Friendship circle gets selective,
You become stubborn and elective.

The end of teens looks umpteen,
When you really cross nineteen.

Books and academics bring no pleasure,
Opposite sex, dance and music is treasure.

6. The Adulthood

On crossing the age of twenty and one,
You reach a stage full of frolic and fun.

Adulthood is in full frame,
Arrogance is the second name.

You simply become more arrogant,
You walk, talk, sleep and act errant.

You walk arrogantly, you talk arrogantly,
You stand arrogantly and sit arrogantly.

You eat arrogantly, you sleep arrogantly,
Only with opposite sex you conduct gently.

Between twenty and twenty five,
You are in your own bee-hive.

You wish to cut short all procedures,
And want to enjoy all worldly pleasures.

You try to push where you have to pull,
And pull where you have to push and mull.

Everything appears simply illogical,
And you try to get and act surgical.

College days are spent roaming,
Studies are off and you get storming.

Suddenly you realize time is gone,
Then you try to struggle alone.

No knowledge, no job and no money,
Then you realize the importance of time honey!

Then you try to reconcile fast,
Probably the opportunity has gone past.

Idealism suddenly gets into you head,
But performance and sincerity is dead.

If a girl then parents are a worried lot,
Your marriage and dowry creates worry of sort.

If a boy then you ask all if and buts,
Parents still think you have gone nuts.

Slowly you seek asylum with vices,
Fags, liquor, romance and spices.

You try and hunt for a job,
You also try to simply hob-Nob.

The new pleasure called sex,
Suddenly knocks at the apex.[10]

You spend time, effort and money,
To search and organize for a honey.

Without realizing the time and loss,
Frolic and fun you tend to engross.

From arrogance you turn to romance,
Start liking pubs, disco and dance.

Speed with cars, scooters and bikes,
Girls, Guitar and roaming on bikes.

To eat drink and make merry,
Dance, drink whiskey and sherry.

The adulthood goes with a bang,
In midst of all vices you hang.

---

[10]Head

7. *The Marriage and Family*

So far you stood young and alone,
With marriage the bachelorhood is gone.

So far so good you stood,
You bore the brunt of adulthood.

Life now begins around twenty six,
With marriage you find in a little fix.

Soon the marriage is finally consumed,
But you get a little drawn and confused.

Was it all for fun and pleasure?
Or your spouse is life's treasure?

As the years get slowly past,
Your physical urges increase fast.

To spouse and beloved you cling,
Career and parents are put at a sling.

After crossing the mark of thirty one,
You start behaving like a flirty one.

This tendency increases with age,
And it becomes embarrassing at this stage.

With physical needs overtaking all actions,
Career and job provide no satisfaction.

You wander, plunder and roam a lot,
Till you finally find a suitable slot.

Slowly you realize the real life pace,
When you find yourself out of race.

At times you feel life is gone and spent,
Without scoring any goal and achievement.

You fail to realize where to start,
And start behaving like an up start.

Then you try to reconcile with spouse,
Try to balance between your job and house.

You find yourself in an empty pool,
Money becomes an important tool.

Money, pleasures and more wealth,
With little care for body and health.

You feel fully done and confused,
With mid life blues fully enthused.

When repeated calls fail to attract,
With forty years of life due to subtract.

Then you try to make both ends meet,
Confused and engrossed in office and street.

8. *Parenting and Maturity*

When life approaches close to forty,
You seem to be getting a bit naughty.

On one side are your family and house,
On the other, the children and spouse.

It's time to take care and not run,
Detach from your own frolic and fun.

Wake up and shoulder responsibility,
With grace, fairness and humility.

Your frolic and fun can be at second place,
Your family should come at the first place.

They ask questions and clarifications,
Your answers do not give satisfaction.

They look for action with perfections,
Where as you find it at dissatisfaction.

They demand for more time and money,
Together they ask for butter and honey.

You look for a little change and spice,
They demand for their time and price.

You try to put off most of the demands,
They continue to give more commands.

Life now tries to pull fifty,
You continue to appear a bit thrifty.

The so called demand and supply gap,
Becomes wide and you get in a trap.

You have to forget your own spice,
Accept their call, if not, pay the price.

Your mind and body do realize,
How you are failing to recognize?

The demand of family, career and wife,
These are called real blues of mid life.

Wake up O' dear hubby and dad,
Before you are called good and bad.

Shoulder thy all responsibilities,
Realize their demands with sensibilities.

Your remainder life is now for children,
Forget about your spice and fun.

This is the time to make up for them all,
So that they can grow big and tall.

Do not shy away from this crucial age,
Try to wake up and make up at this stage.

9. Preparation for Retirement

When you are nearing fifty,
You become a little thrifty.

From now to ten years hence,
You will be on the retirement fence.

Start counting years and savings,
Your problems and all the craving.

If you have slept through out your life,
And didn't take care of children and wife.

If your children are not settled,
Then the life appears totally rattled.

Even if you wake up now,
It may be slightly late now.

Start taking account of things,
Before you reach end of innings.

Settle children and take care of spouse,
And ensure you don't hide like a mouse.

Start planning for a retirement house,
Where you may live with your spouse.

Buy a new and small conveyance,
So that you are not held in abeyance.

Park your savings in such a way,
That savings and pension serve as your pay.

Try to settle in a small town,
Close to original roots or home town.

Make a circle of likeminded Company,
Find a small group to get Old Age Company.

Ensure your health and good hygiene,
As residual life depends upon this scene.

Try to keep away from any attachment,
Prepare for retirement and detachment.

Take to walking, Yoga and make no fuss,
Life will remain healthy and disease less.

10. Retirement and Detachment

Suddenly you reach sixty after a while,
Then you retire and you are called a senile.

You should now practice some detachment,
From family and all worldly attachments.

The process of 'Van Prastha' and separation,
Must begin quietly without exception.

From family and friends do not go far away,
But in the name of God you simply sway.

Nothing will travel with you my friend,
Even your spouse may not last till end.

So for you tried to do for family and self,
Now find some time for God and yourself.

Try to give to society and have not's,
With whatever little you have got.

Time starts running out of frame,
When old age problems try to tame.

Shed all vices and simplify life in house,
Follow a routine along with your spouse.

"Eat to live" is the final word,
"Live to eat" be cut with a sword.

Some say life ends with retirement,
I say it re-starts fresh with retirement.

Stop expecting too much from others,
Give whatever you can to others.

If you have spent some time on retirement plan,
Then the life will go smoothly through this span.

Simply walk, work and meditate,
Don't try to order, expect or dictate.

Listen to your spouse and don't live alone,
Live happy, healthy and let the bygones be gone.

11. Sanyas and Godly Attachment

Now you have enough time to pray,
In the name of God Almighty you sway.

Get up much before sun rise,
Have a set routine as per your life size.

Get set for exercise and Yoga mode,
Have two hours regime in this mode.

Take to meditate and shed your laziness,
No poking your nose in others business.

After kingly breakfast, set your pace,
For day's routine and not for a race.

Have princely lunch and rest a while,
Then set yourself for an afternoon trial.

Walk, play, meet people and do social job,
Then return home for evening Hob-Nob.

After evening bath, meditate again,
Minimum one hour without any pain.

Early supper and then early to bed,
Will keep you healthy and on the tread.

Remember 'GOD' and upper circuit,
And keeping cool within your nut.

Regular routine will help you a lot,
Plan, therefore, a regular time slot.

Plan and spend your hours twenty four,
With seven hours sleep and no more.

Two hours for mind, body and soul,
With two hours for health and hygiene goal.

Eight hours routine for some social work,
Four hours for friends, family and God's work.

Slowly you get towards Godly attachment,
Slowly you follow the path of final detachment.

12. Death and Departure

Death is sure for all living beings,
With no exception to anything.

After the soul leaves your body,
You become absolute Mr. Nobody. .

Though the spirit travels simply upwards,
But the body travels always downwards.

Near and dear feel very sad,
Friends and foe also feel bad.

Whether you believe it or not,
Death is absolutely sure shot.

Hope you would have reconciled,
Your assets which you have piled.

Make sure you are just and fair,
In distribution of your money and mare.

Make sure you leave this place,
With equanimity and perfect solace.

Lord Krishna in Geeta has clearly stated,
Think of Him and to Him you are slated.

Think of Him, while departing soul,
And finally you merge in 'Super soul.'

Chapter-7

Guru - God & Spirituality

Modern World recognises India as the land of spirituality. All our so called different religions accept that there is a Supreme Spiritual Power which runs this universe. Some of our religions which do not recognise the theory of God recognize human being as a spiritual entity. They preach that every human being is element of some spiritual power which resides in a human being and every human being is capable of that realization of self and that super power.

The Vedic theory of three Gods, the Creator (Brahma), the Preserver (Vishnu) and the destroyer (Mahesh) have shown their presence in India/ Himalayas and they are worshiped all over the world in some form or the other. The most modern religion, Sikhism, talks about One God (Ek Onkar).

The Christian talks about Lord Master, the Islam talks about Allah. There appears to be some unanimity on "One Supreme Power" and we may call it by any name. The world accepts the fact that if there is any possibility of attaining Nirwana/Mukti/ Swarg etc it is only through spiritual path as prophesied by our way of life or philosophy of life.

115

It is, therefore, necessary to know something if not complete about this philosophy. The so called realization of self and then realization of God is believed to be achieved by many methods as under:-

- Bhakti – (Japp, Tapp, Prayeres Mantra naam etc)
- Meditation.
- Yoga Samadhi.
- By adopting a guru and follow the path shown by him.
- Sant Matta (Naam/Updesh/Initiation)

My Sanskara and family background has taught me that there is One Supreme Power which runs the universe and rewards every human being based on his "Karma" as explained in "Holy Geeta". You are born to do your duty (Karma) as expected by the society.

My book is not meant for explaining anything about God, Guru and Spirituality but throwing some light on attaining happiness through spiritual path or methods. As brought out in Preface by me that if you are healthy, wealthy, run a happy family and you are accepted in society with respect then you should be living in 'Swaraga' here only. I am sure there is no proof of Swarag Lok or Salvation from life. But in order to convince yourself that having completed your duty or Karma you should find a guru who can lead to path of spirituality.

Guru

Saint Kabir has said that when we buy an earthen pitcher we see and test it from all possible ways and then only buy it. Similarly you should convince yourself completely and should not leave any iota of doubt before accepting or adopting a Guru, if at all you have decided to do so.

God

I am convinced that there is a Supreme Power which runs this universe and I am also convinced that there is only ONE for all living beings. I am also quite happy if you do not agree with me on this subject but you must be happy to accept that.

I am also convinced to quite an extent that easiest and most logical method of God realization is through self realization. This can be done by meditation. The concept of Yoga i.e. "Pratyahar, Dharna, Dhyan, Samadhi" is the most practical and logical.

Meditation through "Naam/Mantra" given or blessed by Guru can be employed for achieving self realization and ultimately God realization.

Spirituality

Spirituality also includes study of various Granthas, spiritual books, and way of life of religions. This can be done in later part of life say after your retirement. While you are living your life, performing your duty/Karma then follow the tenets of your own way of life or religion. Some of the modern saints like Saint Kabir Das, Guru Nanak Dev Ji, Sant Dadu Ji and Bulle Shah have written fair amount of literature on Oneness of God and his control over the universe.

As of now, at the age of nearing seventy years I am not competent to say anything more on this issue of Guru, God and Spirituality.

Chapter-8

Death, the Last Happiness of Life

(Why die every day. Do aish till you become ash?)

An old Saying.

The surety of death is the last fact of life. In fact there is that famous sentence about surety of death –"As sure as death". Anyone who is born has to die. If you take all precaution and remain physically and mentally active, you will not live forever and ever. In spite of all advances in the medical field, the mortality rate remains one hundred percent. Dropout rate beyond the age of 70-75 is quite high. Only about one percent or so reach one hundred.

If death is sure then why do you continue to make castles in the air even after retirement? There is a story in Mahabharata, "The Enchanted Pool". In this the Pandvas were asked by an angel as to what was the most surprising thing in the world? Four of the Pandvas could not reply to this and had been made unconscious by the angel. However, Yudhistra replied that most surprising thing in the world is that every day we see people dying and departing still we think that we may continue to live forever for some reason. The Pandavas were brought to their senses after this reply.

At this stage of life you should look at breadth of life rather than length of life. It makes one sad to see that all sorts of precautions are enforced on old people. Seventy five year old is not allowed to eat a piece of 'Mithia' on Deepawali as he has high blood sugar or high blood pressure. An Eighty years old person is not allowed to smoke a cigarette which otherwise he has smoked for sixty years. At this stage, he may perhaps be able to indulge only in this much.

What, therefore, is a good death? What are you doing to achieve good death? My personal opinion is that good death is one where one dies in his sleep or one dies without suffering too long in a nursing home or hospital and without making his dependant suffer. Lucky are those who die without application of:-

- A surgeon's scissors.
- A physician's hammer or stethoscope.
- Anesthetist anesthesia
- And curse of family for disturbing their peace and enhancing nursing home bills.

You must find time to think and discuss with your family members as to up to what time you want aggressive surgery or cancer chemotherapy given to you. You must tell them up to what stage of life you want coronary artery bypass surgery or kidney transplant with its entire attendant cost and discomfort. Grapes of old age are not sour but bitter. You have to decide whether you would like to leave your life's saving for your children and grand children or pay to the nursing home. You have to decide whether you would prefer death to dependence on others and hospitalization and sufferings.

My intention is not to scare you. If you have maintained an active life then God may be kind to you but who knows about life, sickness and death? There is an excellent book, The Final Exist, written by Derek Humphery which gives a very good step by step, do it yourself procedure with details, the drugs and dosage, legal procedures to avoid problems concerning police. It has a wonderful chapter on how to organize your last evening.

Are you ready to die? Have you drawn up a proper 'WILL', listed out your assets, are the bank accounts in joint names, do the children know where the locker key is? These are routine matters but what is often not discussed is what should be done if you suffer a stroke which robs you of speech and capacity of clear thought process, or you suffer brain damage in an accident. Till when do you want life support to be given? At what stage and by whom can the plug be pulled? One can draw up what is called a living 'WILL' and spell all this out. Otherwise the doctor continues in the name of treatment, the relations do not have the guts and the nursing home bills mount in spite of everyone knowing the final outcome. A word about terminal care is essential. A patient with advanced cancer or terminal kidney failure is sometimes rushed to the hospital so that he can be given a glucose drip or oxygen or artificial respiration. These things in addition to being useless are also cruel. You stick a tube into the guy's throat just when he wants to say his bye-bye and tell you about his bank account number. Treating death as a normal and natural part of life and allowing a painless peaceful departure is much kinder than dying with tubes in your bladder, stomach and nostrils.

Can I choose to die? When I have terminal cancer and the only thing I have to look forward to is pain from which death is the only deliverance, can I choose death? When we see our pet dog suffering from a miserable illness most of us consider it humans to put it to sleep. We are unwilling to extend, the same humanity to our fellow human beings.

After one is dead, for all practical purposes all that is left is one's dead body. The pity is that humanity refuses to accept the inevitability and finality of death. There is that wish to live on forever and ever. Humanity has thus conjured up various fantasies of life hereafter. He wants to be reborn, go into the final loving embrace of the old man up there and has thought up the details of heaven and hell.

With all these complications of life people are willing to cut each other's throats because my book of fairy tales says something different from your book of fairy tales. It is my fervent hope that humanity will one day grow out of these infantile fantasies just as children grow out of fantasies of Santa Claus or book of fairy tales or just as most of us grow out of ghosts and spirits and that humanity will be able to accept the fact that when one is dead, one is dead! This acceptance is important as it will help one to deal with the death here and now and not to seek escape in some rarefied realms of spiritualism.

Omar Khayyam wrote "I sent my soul through the invisible/ some letter of that after life to spell/ and by and by soul came back to me/And answered I myself are heaven and hell". It is with yourself that you have to make your peace. One has to understand oneself and say well that's me. I do not need any one's permission or approval to be myself. If I do not have the guts to be myself as a senior citizen, I will never have the guts.

Philosophy of Life

Mercifully, life, birth and death are still controlled by that supernatural power or Almighty and it's not in our hands. But having lived well, served well and made your mark in life you would have to decide on the following:-

- You should make peace with yourself and you should now think of dying peacefully.

- You should not make your family run in circles and cause confusion in their life by attending to your sickness when the result of which is mostly known.

- You may like to leave your savings to your children and grand children rather than paying the hefty bills or nursing homes and hospitals.

- You may like to decide in preparing your living 'WILL' and decide up to what time you should be hospitalized.

- You may accept to make the "The Final Exit" as prescribed by Derek Humphrey in case you suffer from any one of the terminal diseases by a stroke of bad luck.

Chapter – 9

Cloud Nine

I have discussed the contents of my book after the original draft was ready, with some of my friends who have suggested some post script. I then discussed these with some of the experts in the field of personal finance management. These issues are looked at again and some suggestions are made thereafter. Before I give out their views, I would like to say that if you are healthy, have reasonable wealth, happy family, acceptance in your society and you are able to remember God, then you are a happy man.

Savings

Budget 2019-20 has brought out some good decisions, specially for the salaried class. These decisions have been analysed by experts and these are likely to affect the savings and investments of salaried class in a big way. However, as far as savings are concerned, it is confirmed that PF/PPF/Service/ Provident Fund is the best saving for the salaried people. It is, therefore, recommended that all salaried people drawing more than ₹25,000/- per month as total salary should put ₹5000/- to 6000/- per month in PF/PPF. In spite of receiving less tax rebate and lower rate of interest, this is the best saving for salary class of people.

Investment other than PF/PPF

It is recommended that the investment which salaried people should make should be in mutual funds which are 'Index related stocks' and Government bonds and debt funds. Free investments with high risk in stocks and shares, specially after retirement, is not recommended being too speculative and high risk management. Salaried class of people have white money and this should be invested in safe and risk free investment. Priority for savings are as follows:-

(a) PPF/PF.
(b) Post office Monthly Income Plan.
(c) Mutual Funds (Index related stocks).
(d) Debt Funds.
(e) Stocks and shares.
(f) Fixed deposits in banks.

Outstanding Loans

Some finance experts recommend that we should retire with no loan liability outstanding against us. Others feel that this may be true for all other personal loans but a housing loan up to the age of 65 years is advantageous to the loanee as it provides fairly good tax relief. The interest paid on housing loan provides relief in showing negative housing income and the principle repaid qualifies for rebate under Sec 88. As far as other personal loans are concerned, I agree with the suggestion that one should retire without any loan liability.

Income Tax

As the rebate in income tax has gone down by nearly 50%, and may go down further, it is further recommended that investments are carried out in post office monthly income plan to get benefit under Sec 80L as investments up to 4.5 lacs are exempted. Every retired person should take maximum advantage in savings which can give relief on income tax up to the age of 60. Thereafter, the exemption under the privilege of senior citizenship will come in handy.

Health

Eating and Drinking Habits

A suggestion has been made that after 55-60 years of age it is very difficult to change one's eating and drinking habits. I have not suggested any major changes but only minor alterations and simplifications in one's diet. As far as drinking is concerned, you have to stop consuming hard drinks and be a social drinker up to 60 milliliter only. Hard drinks should be consumed as medicine. Smoking, by all means, has to be left. Walking and swimming should be made part of the daily routine.

Physical Exercise

One of my friends has suggested that after retirement a person can't engage himself in such a serious physical exercise regime. He has also objected to the fact of "Bhoga being better than Yoga". He is of the opinion that sex should not be recommended in a book like this.

I have suggested a daily routine to keep yourself busy and occupied. The level of physical exercise is purely dependent upon calories intake, state of health and age. By no means, I have suggested that a retired person should undertake two hours of hard and strenuous exercise like a young man! As long as, the required amount of physical activity is maintained, it is quite sufficient.

Sex

As far as sex is concerned, I have said, "healthy sex", which definitely does not mean excessive indulgence. Sex does not mean only physical gratification. It also means share and care, light comments and humorous lighter side talk and also physical contact with your like partner as on required basis. There is an old saying which means that a person continues to think about sex as long as he desires to eat food. By 'Bhog' I mean even a romantic hug (Jaffi and Pappi) satisfies you as much as sex at this age.

Social Security

It has been pointed out by one of my well wishers that it is better for a retied and old person to join old age home or such clubs where old people are taken care of. This may be alright if you are alone and have unfortunately lost your spouse. You should allow your children the freedom and privacy of living by themselves.

If God has been kind and you are fortunate enough to live happily with your spouse, at this stage of life, and then there cannot be a better and a more secure feeling than living in your own home. If you are alone as a bachelor, widower or divorcee then of course, you can take the decision of staying in an old age home or any other place as you desire.

Old age home may be good institutions for our society to take care of old and non dependent people but those facilities should not be a normal place to live in for every retired and old person. The recent developments in senior-living or senior care are laudable. One of my old friends Col A Sridharan has established a brand "Covai-Care" which has very good projects in Coimbatore, Bangalore and Chennai. If a couple or person is healthy and stays alone should move to these facilities to enjoy the last few years of life.

Dr Aloysius LOH's Ten Mantras of Happiness

Life can begin at 60; it is all in your hands! Many people feel unhappy, health-wise and security-wise, after 60 years of age, owing to the diminishing importance given to them and their opinions. But, it need not be so, if only we understand the basic principles of life and follow them scrupulously. Here are ten mantras to age gracefully and make life after retirement pleasant and happy.

1. **Never say I am aged:-** There are three ages, chronological, biological, and psychological. The first is calculated based on our date of birth; the second is determined by the health conditions; the third is how old we feel we are. While we don't have control over the first, we can take care of our health with good diet, exercise and a cheerful attitude. A positive attitude and optimistic thinking can reverse the third age.

2. **Health is wealth:-** If you really love your kith and kin, taking care of your health should be your priority. Thus, you will not be a burden to them. Have an annual health check-up and take the prescribed medicines regularly. Do take health insurance coverage.

3. **Money is important:-** Money is essential for meeting the basic necessities of life, keeping good health and earning family respect and security. Don't spend beyond your means even for your children. You have lived for them all through and it is time you enjoyed a harmonious life with your spouse. If your children are grateful and they take care of you, you are blessed. But, never take it for granted.

4. **Relaxation and recreation:-** The most relaxing and recreating forces are a healthy religious attitude, good sleep, music and laughter. Have faith in God, learn to sleep well, love good music and see the funny side of life.

5. **Time is precious:-** It is almost like holding a horses' reins. When they are in your hands, you can control them. Imagine that every day you are born again. Yesterday is a cancelled cheque. Tomorrow is a promissory note. Today is ready cash-use it profitably. Live this moment; live it fully, now, in the present time.

6. **Change is the only permanent thing:-** We should accept change – it is inevitable. The only way to make sense out of change is to join in the dance. Change has brought about many pleasant things. We should be happy that our children are blessed.

7. **Enlightened selfishness:-** All of us are basically selfish. Whatever we do, we expect something in return. We should definitely be grateful to those who stood by us. But, our focus should be on the internal satisfaction and the happiness we derive by doing good for others, without expecting anything in return. Perform a random act of kindness daily.

8. **Forget and forgive:-** Don't be bothered too much about other's mistakes. We are not spiritual enough to show our other cheek when we are slapped in one. But for the sake of our own health and happiness, let us forgive and forget them. Otherwise, we will be only increasing our blood pressure.

9. **Everything has a purpose:-** Take life as it comes. Accept yourself as you are and also accept others for what they are. Everybody is unique and is right in his own way.

10. **Overcome the fear of death:-** We all know that one day we have to leave this world. Still we are afraid of death. We think that our spouse and children will be unable to withstand our loss. But the truth is no one is going to die for you; they may be depressed for some time. Time heals everything and they will go on.

"God bless and be Happy".

Appendix

Daily Yoga & Pranayam Regime

Padam Asan

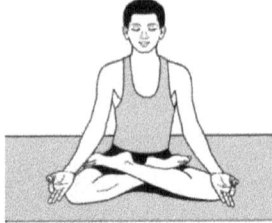

1. Sit in Padam Asan, Yog Mudra or sit in Sukshma Asan for chanting OM. OOoomm should be chanted in such a way that 'O' should be chanted for minimum 10-15 seconds and 'M' for 5 seconds. Om should be chanted after a deep breath in three times and it should be followed by Gyatri Mantar.

2. Then the sequence of warming up by Sukshma Vyam exercise from top to down i.e. Neck, Hand, Legs and Face.

3. After Sukshama Vyam standing run or yogic jogging should be performed for at least 5 minutes.

4. This should be followed by Asanas and then Pranayamas.

1. Manduk Asan (Frog Asan)

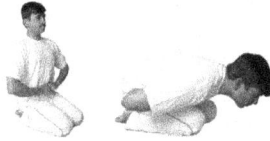

See the picture above sitting in Vajra Asan. This asana is meant to give internal pressure on all the organs of abdominal cavity. Breathe out while bending forward and breathe in while lifting upword. Hold yourself in forward bent position for minimum fifteen seconds. Repeat the bending/lifting at least five times.

This asan is basically a preventive Asan for diabetes, fatty liver and gastric problems. It helps in efficient functioning of digestive system and metabolism.

The asan should be done with empty stomach, empty bladder and bowels clearance.

Manduk Asan

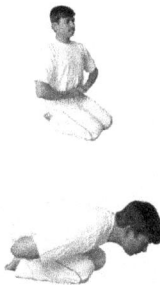

2. Shashak Asan (Heir Asan)

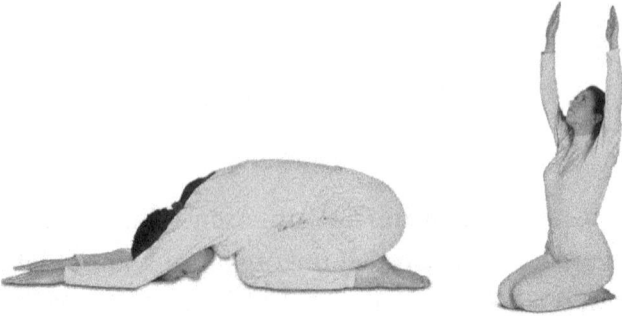

Shashak Asan

See both the picture above. The asan is also performed while sitting in Vajra Asan. The benefits are same as Manduk Asan and breathing sequence is also same.

While bending forward you have to extend your hands as forwards as possible and for head and palms should be touching the carpet. Hold in bent position for minimum 15-20 seconds and repeat this for minimum five times.

This asan should also be done empty stomach, empty bladder and bowels clearance. While lifting upward the hands should extend fully up with biceps touching your ears as shown in the picture.

Shashak Asan

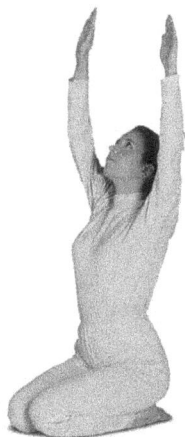

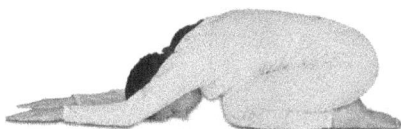

3. Gow Mukh Asan (Cow Face Pose)

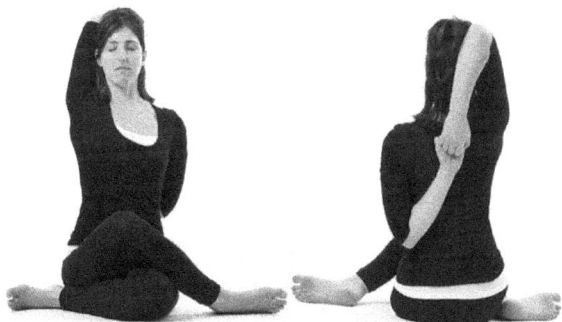

Gow Mukh Asan

See the picture above. You have to sit down with your heals touching the carpet and buttock also resting on the carpet. One leg has to be over the other with knees held in front. Now hold your hands behind your back with same hand being on top position as the leg. If your left knee is resting over the right then your left hand should be up over the shoulder.

This asan is done to prevent shoulder freezing and knee pain. It also helps in preventing and controlling arthritis.

Gow Mukh Asan

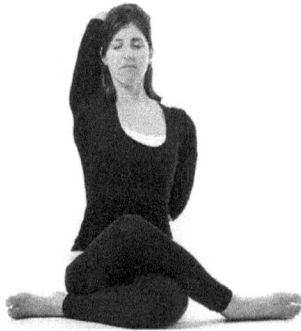

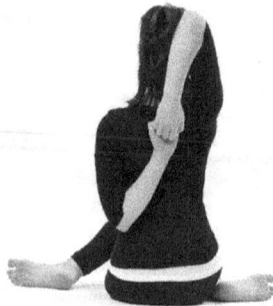

4. Vakra Asan

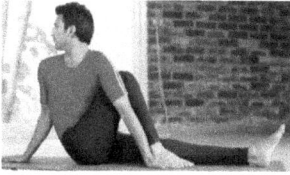 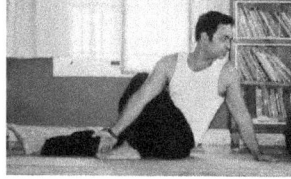

Vakra Asan

This is the last asan is sitting position. See the picture in details. The position of legs and hand is important. The hand behind is opposite of the leg extended in front. The leg which is bent is placed close to the knee of the leg extended. Then upper body and the bent leg are twisted in opposite direction in a manner that bent leg (thigh) is putting pressure on abdominal cavity with sort of squeezing effect.

This asan prevents sciatica pains and helps in flexibility of waist line. It also helps in stomach ailments like gastritis and diabetes.

Vakra Asan

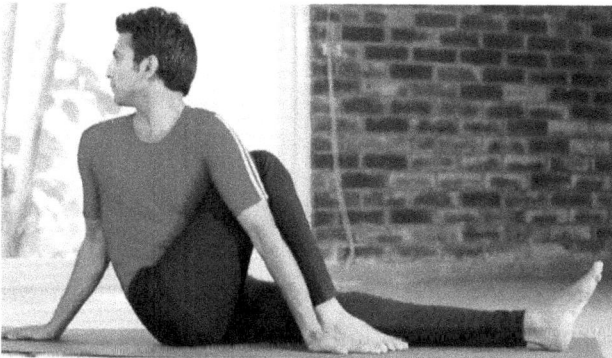

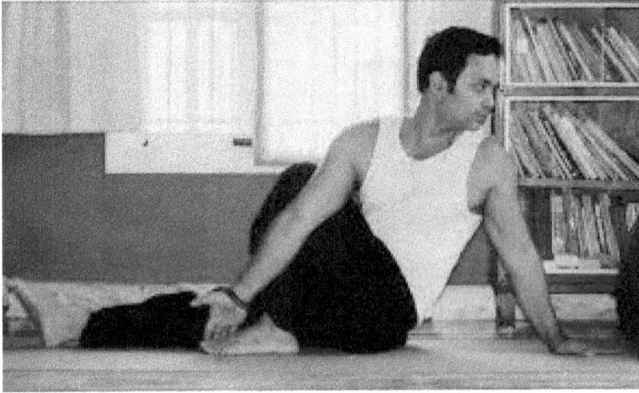

5. Makra Asan

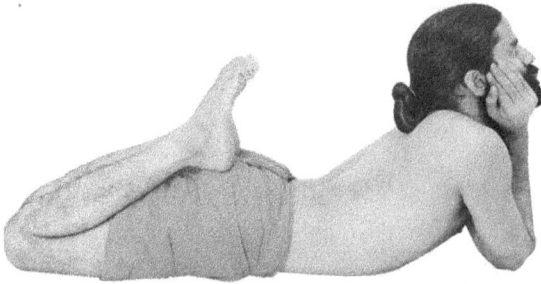

Makra Asan

Next four Asans are in lying on stomach position. If you see the picture opposite both the palms are supporting the chin with elbows placed on carpet close to each other.

Bending of legs so that your heels should touch your hips. First bend your legs attentively at least twenty times and then bend both legs together and try to touch your seat with your heels. Normal breathing should continue.

This asan is meant to strengthen your dorsal muscle and hip muscles to provide strength to your waistline. It prevents sciatica pain and normal low back ache.

Makra Asan

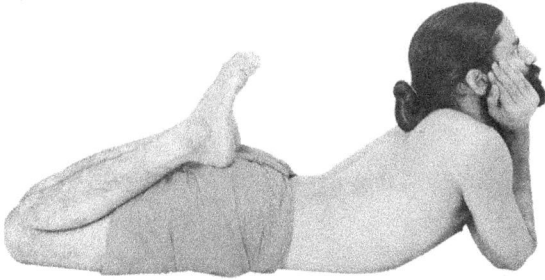

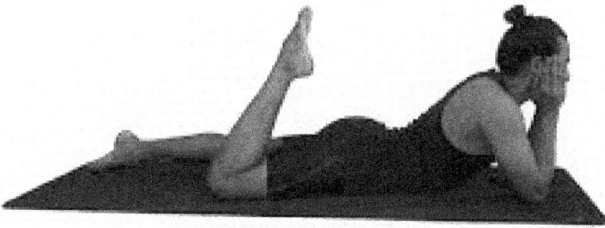

6. Bhujang Asan (Cobra Pose)

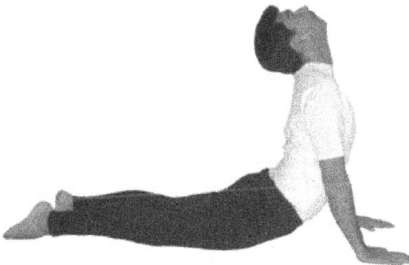

Bhujang Asan

This asan is also performed while lying on stomach position. This has three stages. The first one is lift your trunk with hands up to elbows placed on carpet. The second is with your palms resting on ground and lifting your trunk halfway. The third stage with your palms placed over each other and lifting your trunk fully upward like a Cobra. Breathing in while lifting up and breathing out while coming down. Do it at least ten times. This asan is to strengthen your dorsal muscle and provide strength to all your spinal muscles. It prevents low back ache and sciatica pain. It improves the body posture and helps in maintaining body balance.

Bhujang Asan

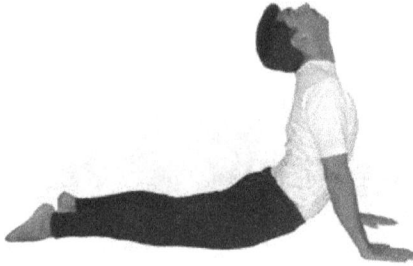

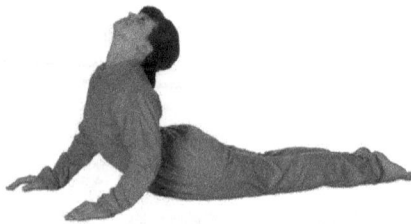

7. Shalbha Asan

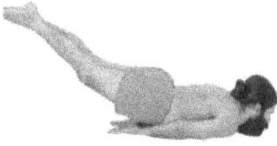 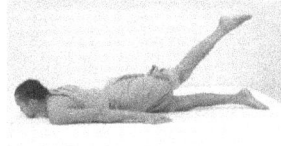

Shalbha Asan

Continue to lie on your stomach. Place your palms under your thighs. Lift your legs upward along with lifting of trunk in synchronization. This asan is in two stages. Firstly lifting your legs alternatively and then lifting them together.

Basically this asan is also to strengthen your dorsal and spinal muscles. It helps in improving body posture and also strengthening lower extremities. This can, in slow speed, be done to reduce sciatica pain.

Shalbha Asan

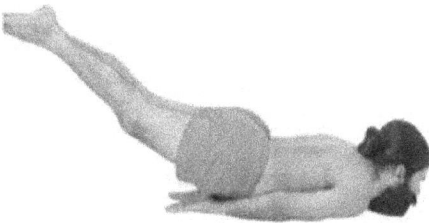

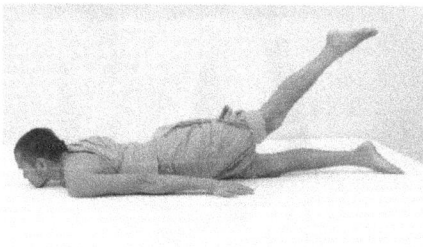

8. Dhanur Asan

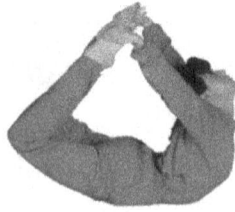

Dhanur Asan

This asan is also performed while lying on the stomach position. This asan is extension of all the three asanas of this group. The aim being to stretch all the spinal and lower extremities joints so that they are stretched fully to remain effective.

This asan also strengthen the dorsal, spinal and leg muscles to enhance blood supply and strength to those muscles. You should be able to hold your ankle and stretch upwards with holding of breath. As you advance in practice you should be able to slowly roll on your stomach by regulating your breath.

As this asan is an extension of first three asanas the benefits of those three asans are also stretched and extended.

Dhanur Asan

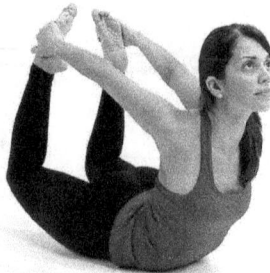

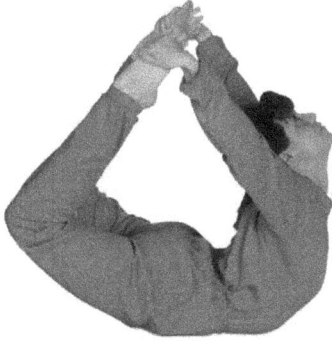

9. Markat Asan

Remaining four Asana are in lying on back position. Markat asan has four stages. Hands are fully extended in line with shoulder and legs are folded with feet together. In first stage you turn your legs together in left direction and the trunk and head in Right directions. Do this slowly for about ten times. Then separate your legs, in folded position, by a distance of one and half foot. Then turn the legs and the trunk as in the first stage. Do it about ten times. In the third stage the legs should be lifted by about six inches in folded position and repeat the bending movement as in stage 1 and 2 at least ten times. Feet should not touch the carpet. Fourth stage is leg fully extended and touching the extended hands.

Breathing should be controlled along with movement of the trunk. Breathe in while your chest is fully extended.

This asan is the strengthening upper legs, buttocks and waistline muscles.

Markat Asan

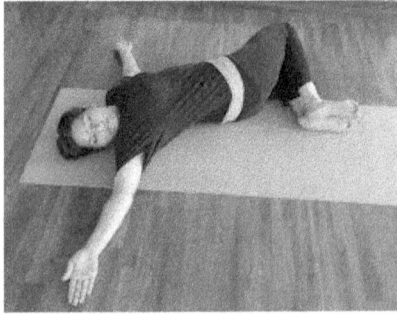

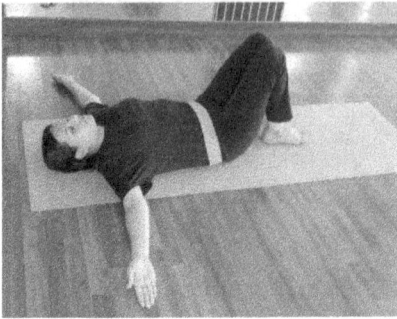

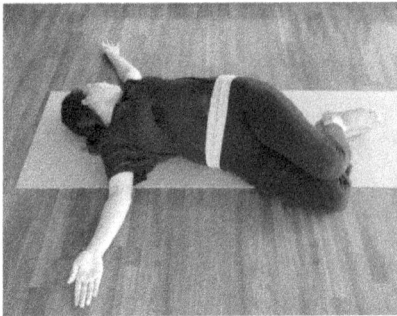

10. Pawan Mukta Asan

This asan is performed in two stages. In stage one you should do it with one leg fully folded with the thigh touching the stomach and knee being touched by your mouth. The second leg should be fully stretched up and extended forward. Repeat this with alternative legs at least ten times each. The second stage is with the both legs folded. Holding both your folded legs tight by locking your hands try to roll on your back smoothly. Be very careful while rolling back not to hit the head on the floor/carpet and try to sit up on your buttocks while rolling forward. If you have spondylitis then do not lift your neck.

This is a very useful asan for all gas related problems. You find that all Apana Vayu (Stomach and intestinal gases) are made to escape through anal canal and you will feel light and charged. This asan is as the name suggests will make you free of gases of the abdominal area.

Pawan Mukta Asan

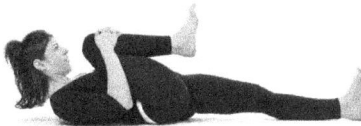

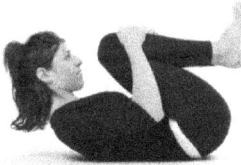

11. Ardhahal Asan

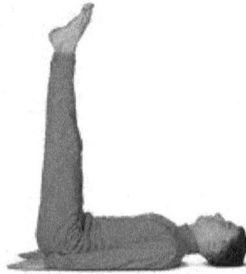

Ardhahal Asan

This asan is also performed while lying on back position. The aim is to exercise and move your legs in all possible directions i.e. cycling forward and rearward, rotating around the hip joint, lifting both the legs in straight position right upto 90 degree to the trunk. Sequence should be:-

- Cycling forward & rearward.
- Rotation of legs individually and then combined.
- Lifting both legs upward and holding them in that position for 2-3 minutes.

This asan is helpful in strengthening the lower limbs waist line muscles and stomach muscles. This is an extension of first two asanas in this position.

Ardhahal Asan

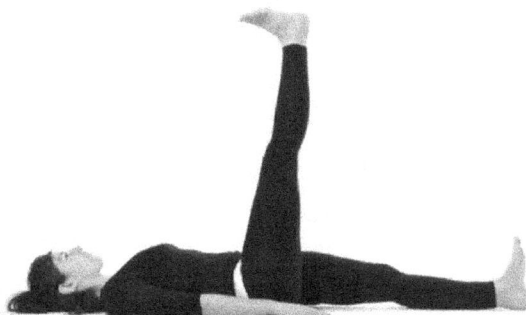

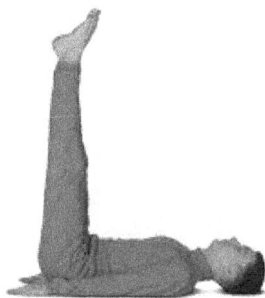

12. Duvi Chakra Asan

This asan is also done lying in the back position. This is opposite of Dhanur Asan. The difference being it is performed on reverse side. There are two methods- firstly, while lying down on your back you lift your body upward supported by hands and legs. See picture. Second method is you bend backwards and land on your hands. This must not be done without the support of an assistant or coach/guide/yoga Asst. There is always a danger of falling back on your head causing serious head injuries.

The benefits are same as Dhanur Asan and hal Asan. Basically this to strengthen the upper Torso, shoulders, dorsal and spinal muscles.

Shav Asan

At the end of 12 Asans lay down like dead body for one- two minutes. Try to feel your body touching every part with the mat and maintain slow speed (8-10) breaths per minute.

Duvi Chakra Asan

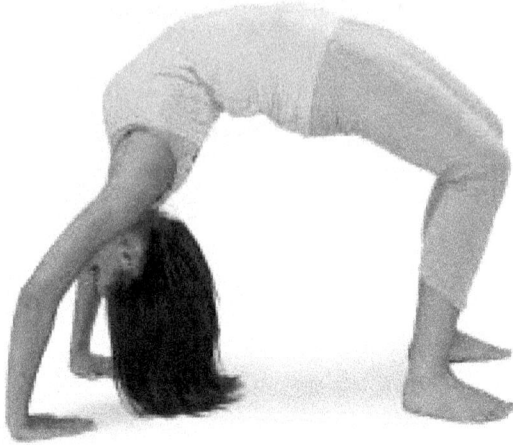

Shav Asan

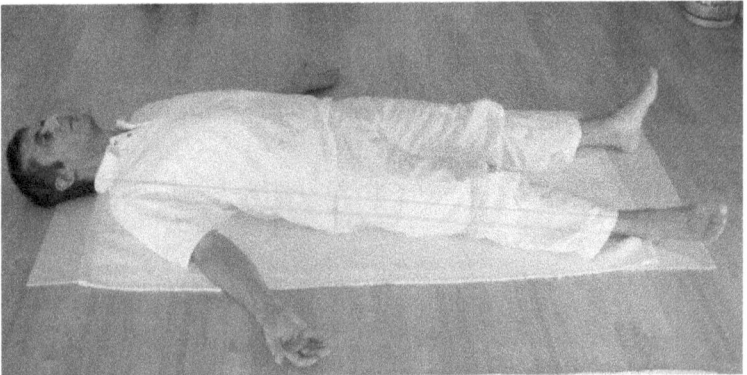

PRANAYAM

Prana is the source of life and when it leaves a human body the clinical death takes place. We generally say that the prana has left the person. There are a total of 16 pranayams prescribed in Grahind Sanhita. **Swami Ramdev Ji** has prescribed a set of **nine pranayams** for daily regime which will give full benefit of health, penance and meditation. These Pranayams are:-

- Bhastrika
- Kapalbhati
- Bahya
- Agnisar
- Ujjaiyee
- Anulom-Vilom
- Brahamari
- Udgeet
- Pranav

In Astang Yog the sequence prescribed is Yam, Nyam, Asan, Pranayam, Pratyahar, Dharna, Dhayan and Samadhi. Pranayams are the foundation of Paratyahar (detachment), Dharna (Concentration), Dhyan (Meditation) and Samadhi (the final union) or realization. Pranayam, therefore, are the most important part of daily "Yog Regime". After Shav Asan for about five minutes one should begin pranayams.

Bhastika Pranayam

- This is also known as deep breathing (bellowing).
- Sit in Padam, Ardh Padam or Sukh Asan with spine being straight.
- Carry on deep breathing in (2.5 to 3 seconds) and breathing out (2.5 to 3 seconds) through both the nostril. No holding of breath at any stage.
- Continue this process for 40 to 60 times in (5 minutes)

Benefits

- This Pranayam helps in extending breathing capacity. Helps in improving reflexes in sports person, shooter, children and flying pilots.

Cautions

Persons suffering from high BP, hear problem recent surgery in chest and abdomen and epilepsy should do this pranayam with caution. They should not exert, follow slow speed and the length of breath should be controlled.

Bhastika Pranayam

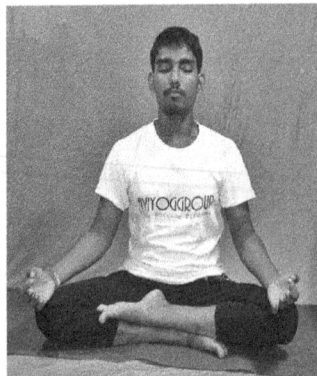

Kapalbhati Pranayam

This pranayam has been called a sort of 'Maha Pranayam' and found most useful for daily regime. It means that kapal i.e. forehead should get a shine by doing this pranaym. You should:-

- Sit in Padam, half Padam or Sukh asan.
- Keep your eyes in mudra i.e. half to full close.
- Employ your abdomen and diaphragm to exhale with force so that you literally hit the breath on your kapal (forehead)
- The frequency is 50-60 breaths in one minute i.e. 250-300 times in five minutes. Total time 17 minutes with one minutes break after very five minute.

Benefits

- Best for detoxification.
- Helps in improving reflexes.
- Enhances energy level.
- Helps in melting abdomen and waiste line fat.
- In woman it helps in opening of fallopian tubes.
- Enhance concentration and thus helps in slow/down syndrome.
- Reduces body tiredness.

Cautions

- Faster rate than 60 per minute can cause high BP.
- Recent surgical cases (upto 3 months) should not practice.
- High BP and heart problem patients should do this with slower rate i.e. 25-30 per minute.

Kapalbhati Pranayam

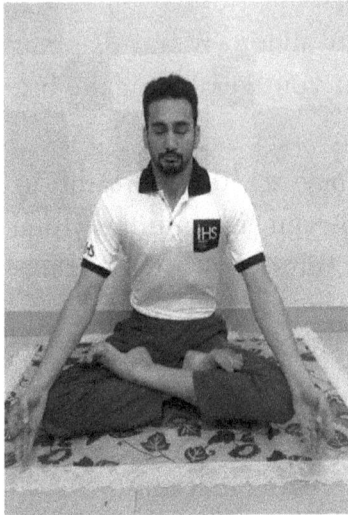

Bahya Pranayam with three Bundhs:

(External Pranayam with three stoppages). This is also called external holding of breath and application of three stops i.e. Mool bandh, pulling of anus upword and closing it, pulling of stomach towards spine and putting Jalandhar bandh and finally closing the respiratory canal (Udyan bandh) by putting chin on the chest. The process of holding and pulling should begin with bottom upword and releasing in should be top bottom. Holding out of breath is recommended for minimum 20-30 seconds and maximum for one minute. Continue to sit in Padam, Aradh Padam or Sukh Asan and repeat this two to three time.

Benefits:

- Helps in enhancing energy level.
- Helps in improving digestive power.
- Enhances reflexes and thus makes you alert.
- Helps in controlling diabetes and reducing belly fat.

Cautions:

Person with high BP, heart disease, undergone surgery in any abdominal or pelvic disorder should avoid doing this asan.

Bahya Pranayam with three Bundhs:

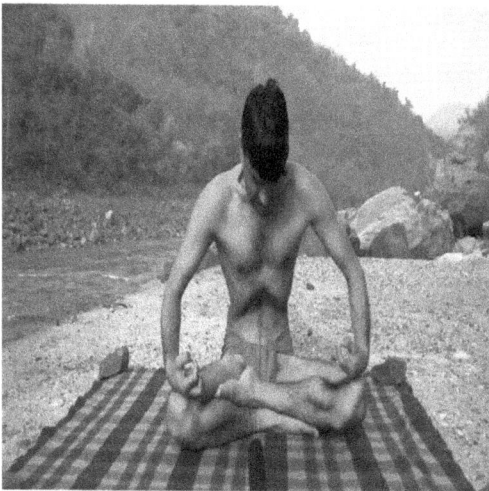

Agnisar:-

(Enhancing Digestive fire). This pranayam also involves in holding out of breath and moving of abdominal muscles forward and near, while sitting in the same pose. You breathe out through your nostril, holding your breath out and move your stomach muscles forward and backward. You would feel the complete shaking out abdominal cavity. Move your stomach muscles 20-25 times while holding your breath out.

Benefits:

- Enhances digestive and metabolic process.
- Reduces abdominal fat.
- Thinning of waist line by reducing all round fat.

Cautions:

Person having undergone abdominal surgery or pelvic distended disease should avoid this pranayam.

Agnisar

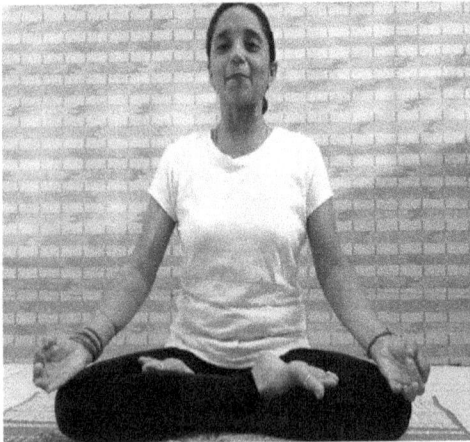

Ujjaiyee Pranayam

This pranayam is basically done for activating the thyroid gland. Sitting in the same pose you breathe out fully through both your nostrils and then breathe in through your nostrils by application of full (breathe-in) force and thyroid gland. Once you have completely breathed in then hold your breath for 20-30 seconds. Breathe out through left nostril while blocking right nostril. This pranayam is recommended for patient's having thyroid problems. It is both preventive and promotive in application.

Ujjaiyee Pranayam

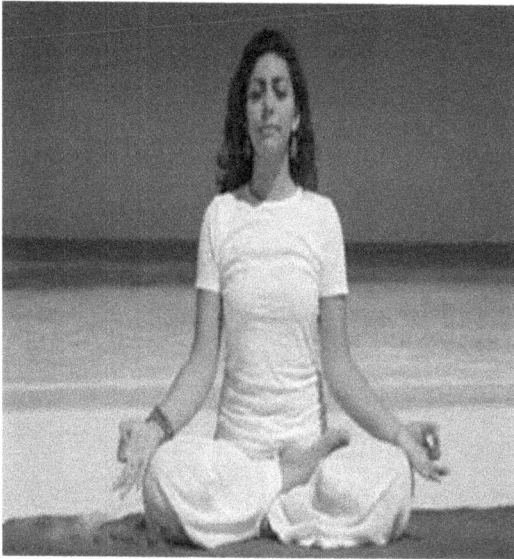

Anulom-Vilom:-

(Alternative Nostril breathing). This is as important as Kapalbhati and it is also called Maha Pranayam. When you are short of time and restricted place it is recommended that you should at least practice these two (Kapalbhati and Anulom-Vilom) pranayam daily.

- Sit in Padam, Ardh Padam and Sukh asan withs spine erect.
- Place you Right thumb on right nostril and ring and little finger on left nostril.
- Breathe in deep by left nostril while blocking right nostril.
- Now block the left nostril and breathe out deep form right nostril.
- Do not hold or stop breathing but continue smoothly. If your hand gets you can change your hand.
- Repeat this cycle minimum 40 to 60 times. (10-12 minutes).
- Breathe in (minimum 3 seconds) and breathe out 2.5 to 3 seconds.

Benefits

- Reduces Blood Pressure.
- Helps in normalization of BP.
- Enhances retaining power or memory.
- Enhances concentration.
- Enhances muscular strength.
- Enhances length of breath thus helps in swimming, running and climbing.
- Helps in high altitude functioning.
- Enhances energy level.

Cautions:

This is considered a safe pranayam. Even after a surgery (one week). This pranayam can be practiced with slow speed and smoothness.

Anulom-Vilom

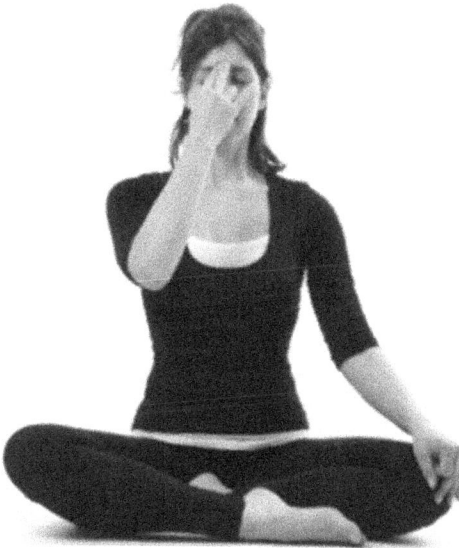

Brahamari Pranayam:-

This pranayam is basically designed to improve the psychological (mental) functions of a person. Brahamari means Bhanwara (bumble bee) which make a specific humming sound. The procedure is:-

- Sit in Padam, Ardh Padam or Sukh Asan.
- Keep your eyes closed and spine erect.
- Place your both hands on your face in such a way that index fingers are on the fore head and three fingers

on eyes. Place your thumb on small ears and block your ear holes.

- Continue the breath normally initially.
- Now take a long breath in and touch your tip of the tongue on the pallet.
- Now breathe out slowly by making a bumble bee like sound (humming sound) slowly by bringing your vocal cords together.
- Breathe in long through nose again and repeat the humming sound. Breathe out should be extended up to 20-30 seconds.
- Repeat the process 7-9 times. You will feel as if you are sending vibrations to your brain lobes.

Benefits:-

- Regulates the pulse rate.
- Helps in improving endocrinal functions.
- Reduces anxiety, tension, depression and stress.
- Helps in fighting examination fever or anxiety.
- Helps in fighting state of Nervous and state of panic.
- Helps in cooling down, maintaining psychological balance and enhancing emotional intelligence positively.

Cautions:

This pranayam is also considered university safe and can be practiced in any state.

Brahamari Pranayam

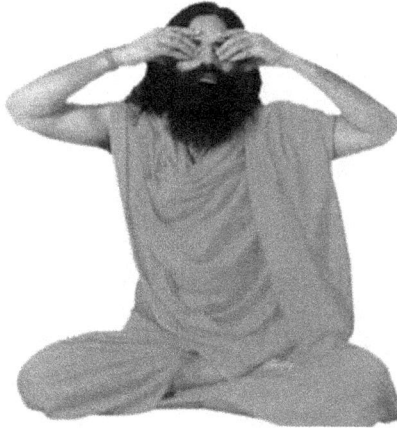

Udgeet:- (Chanting of God's Song/Name)

This pranayam is designed and practiced while chanting Om as under:-

- Sit in Padam, Ardh Padam or Sukh Asan.
- Keep your spine and neck erect.
- Keep your eyes in mudra i.e. nearly closed.
- Take a long breath in through your both nostrils.
- Now chant Om in such manner that 'O' is chanted for 10-15 seconds and 'M' is chanted for 5-10 seconds.
- Chanting of Om should be smooth and in one exhale cycle.
- Repeat this three times.

Benefits:

- The benefits are in line with Brahamari Pranayam.
- Reduces pulse rate.
- Enhances length of the breath.
- Reduces breath rate.
- Helps in concentration.
- Reduces anxiety, stress, tension and depression.
- Helps in maintaining psychological balance.
- Helps in enhancing spiritual and emotional intelligence.

Udgeet

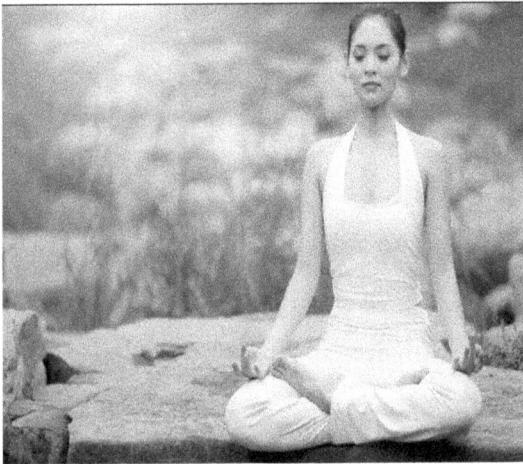

Pranav (Dhayan/Meditation):-

This is meditating pause which is performed in continence of Brahamasi and Udgeet. You concentrate on Sushmama Centre i.e. the area of third eye or centre forehead between eye brows. Try to observe your slow and steady breathing in and out and putting your roaming mind at rest. This helps in meditating and meditation has many benefits as listed below. This should last minimum one to two minutes and maximum 5-10 minutes. Benefits of meditation are:-

(i) **Physiological benefits**

1. It lowers oxygen consumption
2. Decreases respiratory rate
3. Increases blood flow and slows the heart rate
4. Increases exercise tolerance
5. Leads to a deeper level of physical relaxation
6. Builds self-confidence

(ii) **Psychological benefits**

7. Increases serotonin level, influences mood and behavior
8. Resolves phobias and fears
9. Helps control own thoughts
10. Helps with focus and concentration

(iii) **Spiritual benefits**

11. Helps to keep things in perspective
12. Provides peace of mind, happiness
13. Helps to discover your purpose
14. Increased self-actualization
15. Increased compassion
16. Spiritual growth.

Pranav (Dhayan/Meditation)

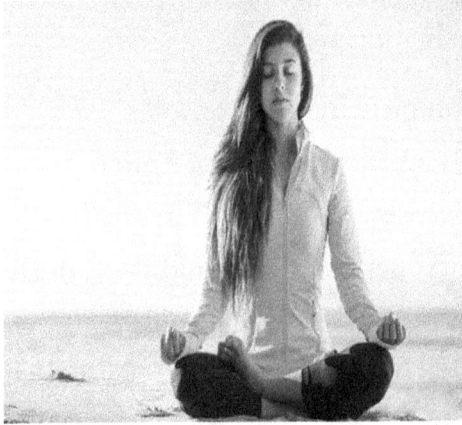

Chanting Om three times to thank God at the end.

About the book

Ultimate Happiness, originally titled as Health, Wealth and Happiness, is all about human needs and how a person can remain happy going through life. How a person can maintain good health and how he can earn and maintain reasonable wealth? In addition to Health and Wealth, other elements which provide happiness to a person are happy family, place in society and mental peace.

- Generally, we run after wealth and spoil our health.
- Then you spend your hard earned wealth to regain your health.
- Health and Happiness can't be bought with wealth.
- It is a vicious circle and a good balance has to be maintained to attain happiness, mental peace and satisfaction.

I am sure the reader will find it quite interesting to read all these issues and finally be Happy, Healthy and Wealthy.

Author